Understanding Public Health

Offering a concise yet comprehensive overview, this textbook explains the fundamental concepts and frameworks that underpin the field of public health. Chapters define key terms and cover topics such as measuring health, technology, equity, leadership, health systems and reform. Real-world health issues, including COVID-19, obesity, HIV/AIDS and climate change, are used to make abstract ideas more easily digestible. Designed for students and professionals interested in public health, it includes learning objectives, illustrative examples, summaries of key takeaways, and comprehension and discussion questions to aid navigation and learning. An instructor manual and test bank are available as supplementary resources.

Julio Frenk is the Chancellor (President) of the University of California, Los Angeles (UCLA) and a globally recognized public health physician and leader in higher education. He previously served as President of the University of Miami and Dean of Harvard T.H. Chan School of Public Health. As Minister of Health in Mexico from 2000 to 2006, he reformed the nation's health system, expanding access to health care for millions. He founded Mexico's National Institute of Public Health and has held top positions in the World Health Organization and other global institutions. His scholarly production includes close to 200 articles in academic journals, as well as many books and book chapters. He has received numerous awards, including the Clinton Global Citizen Award, the Yale Bouchet Medal for Outstanding Leadership and the Welch-Rose Award for Distinguished Service from the Association of Schools and Programs of Public Health.

Claire Chaumont is a public health specialist with over two decades of experience working across more than 15 countries at the intersection of research, policy and practice. Her expertise spans complex health challenges, including global health governance and the connections between health, climate, food systems and commercial determinants. She currently serves as Special Advisor on Strategic Plan Initiatives to the Chancellor at UCLA, where she guides the implementation of the university's 2023–2028 Strategic Plan, and she is also an Adjunct Assistant Professor in the Health Policy and Management Department. Prior to these roles, she helped launch a new department at the World Health Organization focused on strengthening country-level implementation. A Fulbright scholar and political scientist trained at Harvard University, Sciences Po and the London School of Economics and Political Science, Claire has advised governments, multilateral organizations and non-governmental partners, and contributed to numerous policy reports and initiatives that translate evidence into actionable public health solutions.

Suerie Moon leads the Global Health Centre at the Graduate Institute of International and Development Studies in Geneva, where she is also Professor of Practice in International Relations and Political Science. She is a globally recognized expert who has made foundational contributions to the study of global governance and health. She focuses her empirical research on how to achieve more globally equitable innovation and access to medicines, and to strengthen the global governance of outbreaks. Her scholarly contributions include over 70 articles in peer-reviewed journals, 14 book chapters and dozens of reports. She conducts training and other capacity-building activities on global health diplomacy and governance. She also advises governments, intergovernmental organizations and non-governmental organizations, serves on various national and international expert committees and speaks regularly at conferences and with print, radio and television journalists on global health issues.

"As the field of public health faces unprecedented challenges from evolving threats, the need for the development of a conceptual guide for action is great. *Understanding Public Health* arrives at just the right time, delivering a powerful guide to systematic thinking about how new ideas can be translated into effective actions that meet the moment."

Christopher Borick, Lehigh University

"This book is truly a text for the twenty-first century. The systems and determinants approach reflects best practice and underlies the knowledge base needed by today's students if they are to become future public health professionals and decision-makers. The context of public health is changing rapidly and future challenges will require the technical, intellectual approach this text offers, illustrated through the COVID-19 case study. In short, this textbook will serve as an important asset in training students in public health thinking that they will come to rely upon throughout their future career."

Rebecca Fanany, CQUniversity

"Frenk, Chaumont and Moon offer something rarer than another survey of the field: a textbook that treats public health, first, as a way of thinking. By defining the field through its level of analysis rather than its sector or its tools, *Understanding Public Health* gives readers a framework supple enough to hold what we actually do, from the determinants of health to the architecture of health systems, closing with a careful reckoning with COVID-19."

Sandro Galea, Washington University in St. Louis

"This authoritative textbook provides a comprehensive introduction to public health, encompassing the global and the local, and the definitional, conceptual, classification and measurement challenges. Particularly notable is its breadth, from health determinants, viewed historically, through the organized response in the form of health systems, to policy processes and the exercise of power, and finally leadership practices."

Anne Mills, London School of Hygiene and Tropical Medicine

"*Understanding Public Health* offers a clear macro perspective on health systems, grounded in robust frameworks and how systems can improve. It shows how population health and health equity can be advanced through action on determinants, prevention, health promotion and health services, helping students understand the system as a whole, not just its individual programs."

John-Arne Røttingen, Wellcome Trust

Understanding Public Health

Clear Thinking for Effective Action

Julio Frenk
University of California, Los Angeles

Claire Chaumont
University of California, Los Angeles

Suerie Moon
Geneva Graduate Institute

CAMBRIDGE
UNIVERSITY PRESS

CAMBRIDGE
UNIVERSITY PRESS

Shaftesbury Road, Cambridge CB2 8EA, United Kingdom

One Liberty Plaza, 20th Floor, New York, NY 10006, USA

477 Williamstown Road, Port Melbourne, VIC 3207, Australia

314–321, 3rd Floor, Plot 3, Splendor Forum, Jasola District Centre, New Delhi – 110025, India

Cambridge University Press is part of Cambridge University Press & Assessment, a department of the University of Cambridge.

We share the University's mission to contribute to society through the pursuit of education, learning and research at the highest international levels of excellence.

www.cambridge.org
Information on this title: www.cambridge.org/highereducation/isbn/9781009556439

DOI: 10.1017/9781009556392

When citing this work, please include a reference to the DOI 10.1017/9781009556392

First published 2027

Cover image: Credit: CHRISTOPH BURGSTEDT/SCIENCE PHOTO LIBRARY/Science Photo Library/Getty Images

A catalogue record for this publication is available from the British Library

A Cataloging-in-Publication data record for this book is available from the Library of Congress

ISBN 978-1-009-55643-9 Paperback

Additional resources for this publication at www.cambridge.org/UPH.

Contents

Foreword – Gro Harlem Brundtland

In the realm of public health – as in public policy more broadly – theories and frameworks often collide with the sobering realities of implementation. Too often, good ideas never come to fruition. Thoughtless action, though, can be even worse. Clear thinking is essential for effective action.

I should know, having served as Prime Minister of Norway and Director-General of the World Health Organization, and having dedicated my career to sustainable development, global cooperation and health for the last 60 years. I had the distinct honor of being the first public health physician elected as head of government in my country – and also the first woman and the youngest person to occupy such a high office. Given my professional background in science, medicine and public health, it should come as no surprise that during my three periods as prime minister I strove to formulate, implement and evaluate policies on the basis of rigorous evidence.

I was also privileged to have chaired the United Nations World Commission on Environment and Development, whose 1987 report, *Our Common Future*, introduced the concept of sustainable development. Strong evidence served to place environmental issues at the center of the global action agenda.

A decade later, I was elected as the World Health Organization (WHO) Director-General. Among many other initiatives, I led a comprehensive reform of the agency, which included, as one of its cornerstones, the establishment of a new cross-cutting area called Evidence and Information for Policy. Its mission was to develop a firm foundation of scientifically derived evidence both to support the WHO's own technical work and to provide knowledge-based global public goods serving national governments in their efforts to improve the performance of their health systems. There are many examples of the way in which this unit drove the translation of solid evidence into sound policy. Salient among them are the Framework Convention on Tobacco Control, the first ever international treaty established by the WHO; the Global Alliance on Vaccines and Immunization (GAVI), a partnership that is a model of innovative global governance; the Roll Back Malaria initiative, another highly successful partnership; the Commission on Macroeconomics and Health, which served to make health a priority investment for finance ministers, and the first ever comparative analysis of health systems performance in all countries, which spurred a new generation of reforms around the world.

To carry out this ambitious agenda, I recruited an interdisciplinary team of public health professionals, economists, other social scientists, policy analysts, statisticians, data scientists, ethicists and communicators. And, in one more example of life coming full circle, I appointed one of the authors of this book, Julio Frenk, to be the first executive director of Evidence and Information for Policy at the WHO.

Because of my life work, I am delighted to introduce this remarkable textbook, originating from a decade-old course at the Harvard T.H. Chan School of Public Health and grounded in the extensive experiences of its three authors. The book provides readers with a holistic view of what constitutes public health today, questioning its meaning, dissecting our understanding of health and its determinants and exploring the intricacies of health systems and broader systems of health. It also delves into the political and leadership levers that societies can use to enhance health outcomes. In short, this book not only provides a remarkable overview of all aspects of public health, including health systems, but also helps readers to connect those concepts into a cohesive framework, empowering them to see the bigger picture. The ultimate goal is straightforward: to equip readers with the intellectual tools to transform theoretical concepts into tangible solutions adapted to their own contexts.

Our world faces consequential health challenges. Disparities in health care access around the world deprive countless individuals of fulfilling, healthy years of life. The air we breathe, the food we eat and the way we live are making us sick. The rise of artificial intelligence opens a world of possibilities but could just as easily become a nightmare if not managed properly. Climate change threatens to unravel the health gains of the last 100 years and more.

The COVID-19 pandemic underscored the crucial importance of public health, not only in preventing death and illness but also in sustaining economic development, social stability and global cooperation. This unprecedented crisis has raised awareness about the field of public health and attracted more individuals to pursue studies and careers in it. The pandemic has shown that effective public health measures are vital for maintaining the fabric of our societies.

In our era of complex, contradictory and changing problems, the ability to think clearly is paramount. As you embark on this intellectual journey, I encourage you to embrace its lessons with a commitment to action – whether at the international, national or local level. This book provides the conceptual frameworks needed to understand intricate health challenges, but it is you, the reader, who will turn powerful ideas into enlightened action.

Preface – The Appeal of Public Health

A Moment Ripe for Change

In 2020, public health became mainstream overnight. Through an unfortunate but predictable chain of events, a local outbreak of a viral respiratory disease first identified in the Chinese city of Wuhan soon turned into a pandemic, killing millions and durably impacting the lives of billions of people around the globe. In the process, it triggered a confluence of crises with long-lasting economic, social, environmental and geopolitical consequences.

Of course, this was not the first time that public health gained visibility. In recent decades, it has become central to politics in many countries, from efforts to expand health insurance to the growing weight of health care as a sector of the economy. On the global stage, periodic public health emergencies – Ebola, influenza, severe acute respiratory syndrome (SARS) and other diseases – have strained international relations and economic development. And public health has informed essential ethical debates, from how to fight racism and discrimination, to the role of emerging technologies such as artificial intelligence, to social justice and how to care for the most vulnerable members of our societies.

But seldom has the world's attention been so squarely focused on public health. For us, practitioners and researchers of public health, this moment in time is both a challenge and an opportunity. A challenge because public health interventions, if used thoughtlessly or weaponized for political gain, can create more damage than good. An opportunity because renewed interest in public health can stimulate the development of the scientific knowledge and collective resolve required to build a safer and more prosperous future for our interdependent world.

We are in the midst of one of the periods of greatest change in history. Health is undergoing a transition unlike anything humankind has experienced before, which is linked to broader demographic, social and economic transformations and, of course, the looming threat of climate change. The key items of the public health agenda continue to be relevant and urgent: preventing disease, promoting healthy environments and lifestyles, delivering high-quality care to everyone who needs it and protecting families from the financial consequences of ill health, all with the dual objective to pursue social equity and to enable people to live more fulfilling lives. But new elements of complexity have been layered on top of this traditional agenda. We now face multicausal chronic policy failures with no simple solutions, from climate change to the rise of emerging infectious diseases around the world, to the vexing problem of hunger and malnutrition in a world of abundance, to the seemingly intractable imbalances and gaps that constrain the performance of health systems. At the same time, persistent inequality, erosion of social cohesion and the rise of nationalist populism, with its accompanying withdrawal from global cooperation, all weaken our ability to effectively act together on those contradictory and changing problems. In the face of those complex challenges, we are convinced public health will, once again, prove its capacity to respond effectively by advancing understanding that guides action.

Further progress in public health will require a sustained effort to supersede the siloed approaches that limit the effectiveness of both research and professional practice. The antidote to such fragmentation is integration. A first level of integration must occur across disciplines. Already, the most exciting advances in science are taking place at the intersections of traditional disciplines, as exemplified by the creative convergence among the natural, social and data sciences. But we need to go further. There is also a need to integrate across levels of analysis, so that we may examine specific health problems from the genes to the globe. Another domain of integration is between the values of excellence and relevance, which means that while we pursue the highest standards of scientific rigor, we also propose solutions to the most pressing health challenges of our times.

Building the Intellectual Field of Public Health

To address these challenges, there must be a clear conceptual framework that articulates what public health is and what it can do. The aim of this book is to propose such a framework.

Of course, this effort builds on and consolidates a vigorous academic tradition that underpins the creation of new knowledge and guides its practical applications (Frenk, 1993a). Many generations of public health researchers, educators and professionals have made essential contributions along these lines. Like all living traditions, this one should involve a continuous process of renewal.

To guide such a process, it is useful to consider that the development of an intellectual field is based on four elements, which constitute what could be called the "circle of knowledge" (as shown in Figure 0.1):

1. **Conceptual foundation:** Any effort to establish a specific field of research, education and practice must start by establishing its boundaries. Hence, this element involves rigorously defining what constitutes public health. Of note, concepts themselves are subject to change, based on new evidence or learning emerging from the three subsequent steps of this cycle of knowledge, which can lead to a revision of existing paradigms and definitions.

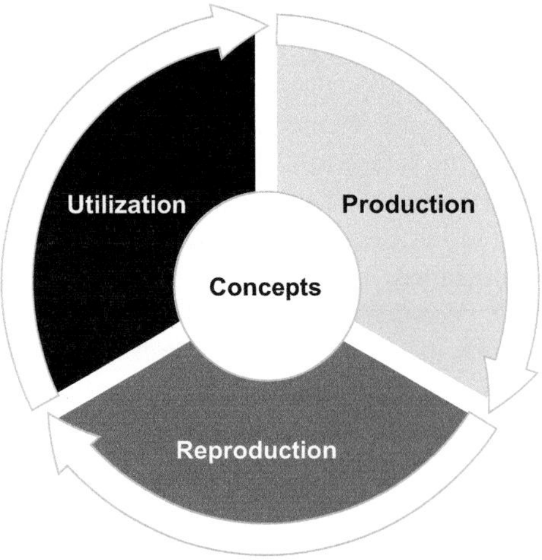

Figure 0.1 The circle of knowledge, showing the conceptual foundations that underpin its production, reproduction and utilization. Adapted from: Frenk J. The new public health. *Annual Review of Public Health*, 1993, 14, 469–489.

2. **Production of knowledge:** The value of public health to society is anchored on an organized effort to produce new knowledge. This element refers to the set of institutions, including schools and institutes of public health, where a critical mass of researchers and professionals come together to generate, through research, the body of knowledge that gives substantive content to the intellectual field.
3. **Reproduction of knowledge:** This element ensures the consolidation and continuity of the intellectual field – and thus the construction of an authentic tradition – through three principal vehicles for reproducing knowledge: educational programs to develop new professionals and researchers, publications to disseminate results and associations for the exchange of ideas and the aggregation of interests. To produce relevant information that takes into account the complexity of today's world, schools and programs of public health need to continuously look outside their walls, at the changing character of their environment, and inside to renew their own organizational structures (Frenk, 1988a).
4. **Utilization of knowledge:** For scientifically derived knowledge to be used, it must first be translated into two types of products: concrete technologies, such as drugs, vaccines, devices and algorithms, and evidence that can guide decision-making based on research results by individuals, professionals and policy-makers. Once it is translated, knowledge can be utilized to provide goods and services to society, including public health services. When knowledge is thus applied, reality is transformed, which generates the need for new knowledge production, thus restarting the circle again. Even though many academic institutions engage in knowledge translation, the final step of applying such knowledge is typically carried out by other organizations in the public and private sectors. Utilization of knowledge by society is of great importance for providing feedback to the individuals and institutions involved in its production and reproduction.

We will not elaborate further on the production, reproduction and utilization of knowledge, as these concepts are discussed in depth by Frenk (1993a). Our key point is that these elements of the circle of knowledge can only be developed if there is a clear conceptual understanding – which is precisely the focus of this book.

From Ideas to Action

Developing a conceptual basis for public health is not merely an intellectual exercise. To the contrary, this book is intended to bridge the gap between ideas and action, to enable readers to develop a rigorous and systematic way of thinking about public health as a guide to action. The fundamental premise of this book is that **clear thinking is a requirement for effective action.**

The dichotomy between thought and action is an expression of the Cartesian divide between mind and body. Yet there is no gap between these two worlds. Ideas are part of reality, and we need them to guide our actions. In turn, practice generates knowledge that, when systematized, can nourish the production of new ideas. This integrative perspective was aptly expressed by Avedis Donabedian, the founding father of the field of health care quality (Donabedian, 1986):

> ... the world of ideas and the world of action are not separate, as some would have us think, but inseparable parts of each other. Ideas in particular are the truly potent forces that shape the tangible world.

Those of us who practice public health aspire to be agents of change. Transforming reality requires clear thinking. Learning facts is essential but not sufficient; it is just as important to understand a series of frameworks that allow you to approach a particular problem and place it in a view of the world – making it possible to understand the problem and then act on it. Action is not separate from thinking. Making sure we connect them systematically can help prevent thoughtless action.

How to Use This Book

With this book, we would like to invite readers to explore the intellectual and practical riches of public health. By laying out the conceptual underpinning of public health, we hope to empower policy-makers, practitioners, students, activists and members of the larger public to thoughtfully and effectively respond to critical challenges.

The book should be of value to anyone interested in public health or intent on making sense of the present moment. In particular, it should appeal to all those working in or studying to join the health professions. It was initially developed around the lectures of a gateway course taught at the Harvard T.H. Chan School of Public Health as a core component of an innovative Doctor of Public Health program, focused on development of leaders. The course has now been taught for nearly a decade, with each edition building upon and updating its content to adapt to a changing environment. In addition, many ideas rely heavily on papers written over the last decades, many with different colleagues.

We hope this book will equip you with an understanding of the foundational concepts that will help to organize your thinking and learning about public health.

The book is organized in 14 distinct chapters, each covering a fundamental public health topic. All chapters include learning objectives at the start, as well as a summary of key points discussed in the chapter at the end. In addition, chapters include comprehension and discussion questions based on the chapter content and designed to be used individually or during class discussions to further understanding of the material.

Supplementary resources are available online at www.cambridge.org/UPH to support instructors in designing their courses. These resources include:

- A comprehensive test bank of questions, organized by chapter, designed to help instructors assess whether students have understood the concepts presented in the book and can apply them in practice.
- An instructor manual, also organized by chapter, which can be used to plan lessons and prepare for lectures and seminars. In addition to the learning objectives, summary of key points and discussion and comprehension questions already included in this textbook, it also includes lesson plans, lecture notes and ideas for class activities and labs.

After completing this book, you should be able to:

- Understand the fundamental concepts underpinning public health as a field of inquiry and an arena for action.
- Relate these concepts to each other through conceptual frameworks.
- Situate specific public health challenges within coherent, integrated conceptual frameworks, in order to facilitate clear thinking about the challenge and effective actions to address it.

- Identify your specific areas of interest and knowledge gaps within a broad, comprehensive view of the field of public health.

The Road Ahead

This book is divided into four sections. Section 1 develops a conceptual framework to define public health. Our goal has been to offer a framework that is coherent and comprehensive, yet also parsimonious. In this spirit we propose that the essential defining element of public health is its **population level of analysis**, in contrast with other health sciences, which focus on the individual and sub-individual levels. Our framework allows us to argue that global health is best understood as an extension of public health, where the population level refers to the entire world.

Alongside its distinctive level of analysis, we propose that public health has two main **objects of analysis**: on the one hand, the health conditions of populations, by which we mean the diseases, risk factors and developmental processes that constitute health status; on the other, the organized social response to those conditions, as it is structured through health systems and systems of health. This distinction is the basis for the next two sections of the book. Section 2 deals with health conditions, their definition, determinants and dynamics. In this section, we explore the link between determinants of health and health equity, and the way recent epidemiological trends and the rise of climate change challenge our traditional understanding of the health transition. Section 3 is devoted to a detailed exploration of health systems, including both the health care and the public health subsystems. In this section, we devote particular attention to the way health systems change, and the political and leadership factors at play to achieve this change. In this respect, the book differs from other public health texts in that we consider research, policy and practice on complex health systems to be an integral part of public health. Along our journey through the chapters in Sections 2 and 3 we explain several frameworks that aim to elucidate the key concepts that underlie health conditions and systems.

Finally, Section 4 ties all the threads together through a case study of the COVID-19 pandemic guided by the conceptual frameworks presented in the preceding sections and some final thoughts on the current context and challenges and opportunities ahead. Throughout the book, we cross-reference the main concepts to the relevant illustrations provided by the pandemic, while also mentioning other practical applications of the frameworks (such as tobacco control, obesity, etc.).

It is our hope that this book will both inspire and clarify: inspire you to pursue the rewarding field of public health and clarify the thinking you need to take effective action in it.

Acknowledgments

Before becoming the book you hold in your hands (or maybe read on your screen), this text took many forms: discussions with colleagues, academic articles, lecture slides and even a barebones pdf of an earlier version that we would share with our students. We are indebted to the many people who made this work possible.

Several chapters in this book are based on previously published articles, some of them with other colleagues. The resulting chapters have all been revised, updated and, in some cases, significantly transformed. We have acknowledged those co-authors throughout the book but want to reiterate here their role in this book's intellectual production. Thanks, in particular, to Avedis Donabedian, Christopher J.L. Murray, José Luis Bobadilla, Octavio Gómez-Dantés, Felicia Knaul, Jaime Sepulveda, Juan Luis Londoño, Rafael Lozano, Tomas Frejka, Tim McDonald and Claudio Stern. More generally, thanks to all the colleagues, mentors, students, editors and readers who have, over the years, nourished our thinking and sharpened the ideas presented in this book.

This book was initially created for a course called "Fundamental Concepts in Public Health," taught to the students of the new Doctorate in Public Health (DrPH) launched at the Harvard T.H. Chan School of Public Health in 2014 to provide advanced education to public health professionals with a focus on leadership development. We are grateful to Sue Goldie, Joshua Salomon and Jennifer Goldsmith, who joined the teaching team at various points over the years and helped strengthen its material. We especially acknowledge the many contributions of Professor Sue Goldie, a leading educational innovator and researcher, who has greatly enriched the original course with a modified format for master's students, while developing new pedagogical resources. Huge thanks are also due to education experts Bonnie Anderson, Erin Driver-Linn, Sejal Vashi and Sirui Wang, who provided invaluable advice on how to improve our teaching approaches, and to our talented teaching fellows, including Kashif Khan, Anshul Kumar, Guilherme Trivellato, Jenny Hsi, Cristina Gago, Kate Wright and Rodrigo Bazua Lobato, who sharpened our thinking and pedagogy with each iteration of the course. We are also indebted to all the DrPH students throughout the years who helped us improve this material with their insightful questions, comments and critiques.

Thanks to our editors at Cambridge University Press, in particular Peter Buckles, Anna Whiting, Tineke Bryson and Jane Adams, who skillfully guided us to ensure this book would be comprehensive yet accessible, as well as 14 anonymous reviewers, who helped improve the text with their thoughtful comments and suggestions. Our deep gratitude goes to Marissa Coppola for her careful research and editing work, which helped get this book to the finish line, as well as Nanette Soto for her amazing work on the pedagogical material which accompanies this book.

Finally, each of the authors thanks the people in our lives who have supported us, helped us grow and make this work possible. For Julio, this includes, in particular, his parents, Silvestre and Alicia; his mentors, Guillermo Soberón, Avedis Donabedian and Rashid Bashshur, and his wife and colleague, Felicia Knaul. For Claire, this includes her family, Catherine, Christophe, Marie, Jean-Baptiste, Jeanne, Etienne, Dea, Louise and Joséphine; her mentors, including but not limited to Suerie and Julio, her many public health friends and colleagues; and finally, her beloved husband Eric Dunipace and baby Aubergine, who, just like this book, took a little longer than planned to see the light of day. For Suerie, this includes her grandmother Illgeum Lee and parents Youjae and Ineon Moon; her mentors, including Julio, Bill Clark, John Ruggie and Ilona Kickbusch; and her family, Chan and Teju Park, who allowed her time and space to think and write even on sabbatical family vacation.

We have dedicated our professional careers to the field of public health because we all profoundly believe that health is key to the well-being and development of individuals and societies. Our recognition goes to all those in the public health community and beyond who strive for a healthier, kinder and more just world and who work tirelessly every day to turn the abstract concepts discussed in this book into improved realities for concrete persons around the world and across generations.

Section

1

Thinking about Health

Chapter 1

What Is Public Health?

Learning Objectives

- Describe multiple concepts of public health and analyze the intellectual and practical implications of adopting different conceptualizations of this term.
- Identify a working definition of public health.
- Relate this concept of public health to scientific disciplines, conceptual frameworks and terms commonly used today.

1.1 Introduction

Public health lies at the crossroads of multiple dimensions: biology and society, individual and community, science and scholarship, evidence and ethics, analysis and action, the local and the global, excellence and relevance. In addition to its intrinsic value, health is a means for personal and collective advancement. It is, therefore, an indicator of the success achieved by a society and its institutions of government in promoting well-being, development, security and social justice.

As a field of knowledge and practice, public health has historically been one of the vital forces that has led to reflection on and collective action for equitable social advancement. In the twenty-first century, and even more so since the COVID-19 pandemic, the field of public health is itself at the threshold of a new era with vast new challenges and opportunities. The global public has seldom been more aware of or interested in providing, as the Constitution of the World Health Organization puts it, "the highest attainable standard of health [which] is one of the fundamental rights of every human being" (World Health Organization, 1946). But at the same time, the health of the planet and its people currently faces unprecedented and daunting obstacles.

Over the next 14 chapters, we will offer definitions of concepts and frameworks that will allow you to think clearly about public health. We will use models as a way of representing, simplifying and managing real life. We must, of course, never think that a model fully captures the multidimensionality of reality. Models are not a substitute for this. Rather, they allow us to handle the world's complexity in a manageable way that can enable our efforts toward enlightened transformation of reality as agents of change. Thinking clearly about what we want to change, and how, is the goal of this book.

The ultimate test of our models' usefulness is whether they will help us take constructive action.

1.2 An Elusive Concept

To start, we must define the term "public health" itself. This term is charged with ambiguous meanings. Throughout its history, five connotations have been particularly prominent. The first equates the adjective "public" to governmental action, that is, the public sector. The second meaning is somewhat broader than this, as it includes not only government programs, but also participation of the organized community, that is, "the public." The third connotation identifies public health with "non-personal health services," that is, services that a specific individual cannot appropriate because they are targeted at the environment (e.g., sanitation) or the community (e.g., massive health education). The next usage expands on the third one, because it adds a series of personal preventive services for vulnerable groups (e.g., maternal and child care programs). Finally, the expression "public health problem" is often used, especially in non-technical language, to refer to diseases or risk factors that affect many people or pose a large threat.

There are also associations among these different meanings. In some industrialized countries, for example, the private sector has tended to provide most personal therapeutic services, whereas the public sector has assumed responsibility for preventive and non-personal services, which tend to deal with high-frequency problems. This has reinforced the notion of public health as a separate subsystem of services provided by the government and parallel to the mainstream of high-technology curative medicine.

Such a limited perspective has led to several attempts at redefining public health. In the face of the profound changes that have characterized human health (which will be further explored in Chapter 6), there have been many proposals to define or redefine public health.

Most often though, these definitions, by trying to reject earlier ones, tend to limit the scope of public health. For example, let's consider the following two definitions.

In 1913, Hibbert Winslow Hill, at that time director of the Public Health Institute of the City of London in Ontario, Canada, gathered in a volume a set of lectures he had delivered the two previous years in order "to present the modern conceptions [of health] to the medical profession and to the public." The title of this volume was *The New Public Health* (Hill, 1913). In 1920 these conferences were revised and expanded, giving birth to a book with the same title (Hill, 1920).

What was Hill referring to when he spoke of the "new public health"? Considering the advances of microbiology a few decades earlier, the "new" was the search for the specific agent of each disease. To leave no room for doubt regarding his adhesion to what Dubos has called the "doctrine of specific etiology" (Dubos, 1959), Hill wrote the following: "... all through hygiene and sanitation specific troubles must be met by specific measures directed specifically against the real specific cause of that trouble" (Hill, 1920). This vision allowed for the individualization of health problems, in opposition to the previous notion that looked for the causes of diseases in the non-specific influence of the environment. Thus, Hill was able to offer the following distinction (Hill, 1920):

> The essential change is this: The old public health was concerned with the environment; the new is concerned with the individual. The old sought the sources of infectious disease in the surroundings of man; the new finds them in man himself.

Sixty-eight years later, in 1988, the British authors John Ashton and Howard Seymour published another book with the title *The New Public Health* – apparently with no knowledge of Hill's contribution, which they don't cite. Now the definition was exactly the opposite of the one offered by what we could call the "old new public health" (Ashton and Seymour, 1988):

> ... [T]he New Public Health goes beyond an understanding of human biology and recognizes the importance of those social aspects of health problems which are caused by lifestyles ... Many contemporary health problems are therefore seen as being social rather than solely individual problems ...

The two contradictory formulations analyzed above show the way in which public health has come full circle in the search for its identity by rejecting its own past. What is needed is a formula to integrate the biological and the social, so that successive notions of public health evolve in an ascending spiral, rather than in a circle. What could be an essential defining criterion for public health that can transcend the changing conceptions of each historical moment?

The remainder of this chapter is precisely an attempt to define the essence of public health.

1.3 The Essence: Level of Analysis

In an effort to supersede earlier contradictions, we propose a more comprehensive conception of public health. According to this view, the adjective "public" does not designate a particular set of services, a form of property or a type of problem, but rather a specific level of analysis: **the population level**. In contrast to clinical medicine, which operates at an individual level, and biomedical research, which analyzes the sub-individual level, the essence of public health is that it adopts a perspective based on groups of people or populations. This population perspective inspires the following definition: public health is an interdisciplinary field of inquiry and a problem-based arena for action focused on health processes and outcomes at the population level (Frenk, 1988b).

It is worth noting that this definition is by nature neutral. As such, it does not carry in itself any particular goal or value, for example, a particular focus on equity or human rights, which can sometimes be implied by definitions focused on particular groups or activities. It merely describes a field of inquiry and action. *How* public health is researched and practiced will then reflect societal values.

We now turn our attention to the way this broad definition impacts our understanding of the scope and boundaries of public health research and public health practice.

1.4 Public Health Research

As an interdisciplinary field of research, public health involves the application of the biological, social, behavioral and quantitative sciences to the study of health phenomena in human populations. Several authors have proposed frameworks for understanding public health. The one we present below encompasses two main objects of analysis: the epidemiological study of the health conditions of populations; and the study of the organized social response to those conditions, in particular, the way in which such response is structured through the health system (Frenk, 1988b; Frenk et al., 1988).

To visualize the role of public health within the more general field of health research, we can relate the levels with the objects of analysis. This produces the typology shown in Table 1.1.

Table 1.1 Typology of health research. Adapted from Frenk (1993a)

Level of analysis	Object of analysis	
	Conditions	**Responses**
Individual and sub-individual	Biomedical research	Clinical research
Population	Epidemiological research	Health systems research

For the first dimension of the typology, we recognize two levels of analysis: one addresses individuals or parts of individuals (i.e., organs, cells or subcellular elements); the other is the aggregate level of groups or populations.

For the second dimension of the typology – the objects of analysis – we define conditions as the biological, psychological and social processes that constitute the health status of an individual or population. Conditions are expressed in specific diseases, risk factors and developmental processes such as pregnancy or child growth. By response, we are not referring to the internal physiopathological reaction to a given disease process, but to the external response that society organizes for improving health conditions. The main vehicle for such a response in modern societies is the health system of each country, although broader "systems of health" are increasingly required to address its complex determinants. (Chapter 14 illustrates the concepts of health conditions and organized social response by applying them to the case study of the COVID-19 pandemic.)

Of note is the fact that behaviors are involved in both health conditions and responses. With respect to the former, individual and family behaviors are powerful risk factors for many diseases, as we will see in Chapter 5, when we analyze the determinants of health. In addition, some mental health conditions have an important behavioral component. Behaviors also feature prominently in the response to health conditions. Very often, the first step of the response is the decision to seek care in the face of symptoms or risks and to comply with provider instructions. Vaccine hesitancy is a relevant current example of the way in which patient behaviors shape the effectiveness of health system responses. Finally, it is important to consider the behaviors of providers, especially in the way they relate to patients, colleagues and their own well-being.

Crossing the two dimensions of levels and objects of analysis yields the three principal types of research that characterize the field of health: biomedical, clinical and public health research (encompassing epidemiological and health systems research). Thus, most biomedical research is concerned with the conditions, processes and mechanisms of health and illness, especially at the sub-individual level. Clinical research focuses primarily on studying the efficacy of the preventive, diagnostic and therapeutic responses applied to the individual. The objects indicated above can also be analyzed at the population level. As shown in Table 1.1, this is precisely what constitutes the two types of public health research: epidemiological research, which studies the frequency, distribution and determinants of health conditions (Donabedian, 1973); and health systems research, which we define as "the scientific study of the organized social response to health and disease conditions in populations" (Frenk and Durán, 1990).

Epidemiological research may, in turn, be classified into two areas of analysis. It is possible to start with a set of determinants to study their various consequences. This is the case with environmental, occupational, genetic and social epidemiology. Or research may instead begin by examining some specific health condition, for example, injuries, infectious diseases or chronic and degenerative ailments, to investigate its multiple determinants.

Health systems research also includes two major categories. The first can be called "research on health systems organization," which is focused on the micro- and intra-organizational level of the health system. It studies the combination of various resources for producing health services of a given quality and technological content. Thus, it includes research on health resources and health services. Health services research is part of health systems research, as it seeks to analyze the primary products of the system: the services. However, the literature still commonly uses the terms "health systems research" and "health services research" interchangeably. The second category of health systems research is called "health policy research." It focuses on the macro- and inter-organizational levels of the health system (Hoffman et al., 2012). Its purpose is to investigate the social, political and economic processes that determine the specific forms adopted by the organized social response. Therefore, it studies the determinants, design, implementation and consequences of health policies (Shi et al., 2009).

To illustrate the distinctions between the four types of research illustrated in Table 1.1, consider the example of tobacco cigarettes outlined in Box 1.1. In this case, the types of research study the health effects of cigarette smoking but focus on different objects and levels of analysis.

Naturally, the typologies proposed here are just abstractions for distinctions that are never so clear-cut in real life. In particular, the four main types of health research shown in the central part of Table 1.1 should not be seen as mutually exclusive. They are connected in many ways. Various fields, such as bio-epidemiology, clinical epidemiology, decision analysis, technology assessment and implementation research deal with interfaces among the four types. Indeed, the principal message of Table 1.1 is integration.

The essential difference between public health research, on the one hand, and biomedical and clinical research, on the other, is not in the objects but in the levels of analysis.

The future of public health will depend largely on its ability to build bridges with the other types of health research and to make its specific and irreplaceable contribution to this analysis at the population level. Thus, the challenge is to integrate levels and objects

Box 1.1 Research on cigarette smoking

Biomedical research might focus on how smoking cigarettes affects lung cells. Clinical research might consider how it affects bodily functions such as breathing, or how effective different interventions are to help a patient stop smoking. Epidemiological research could study the prevalence of smoking across a population or the factors that seem to increase or decrease the prevalence of cigarette use over time. Within health systems research, health services research might examine how to reach groups that have been historically marginalized, or people from lower-income socioeconomic groups, with effective smoking cessation programs. Finally, health policy research (another subset of health systems research) could study the effects of increasing taxes on cigarettes, or implementing higher age restrictions on cigarette consumption.

of analysis so as to achieve a full understanding of the broad health field. In the case of public health, this also requires integration among scientific disciplines.

1.5 The Role of Disciplines

The very definition of public health research involves an effort to achieve interdisciplinary integration. An important obstacle to such integration has been the tendency to identify each level of analysis with a given discipline. In particular, the resultant confusion suggests that the biological sciences are applicable only to the individual and sub-individual levels, whereas the population level is the exclusive jurisdiction of the social sciences.

All human populations are organized into societies, which is why the social sciences are indispensable for fully understanding health in populations, namely, public health. However, there is also a biological dimension of human populations, which is expressed, among other phenomena, in the distribution of genetic characteristics, herd immunity and the interaction of humans with other populations, such as microorganisms. In particular, the field of "bio-epidemiology" encompasses the study of the biological determinants, risk factors and consequences of health processes in populations, as well as the use of methods and techniques derived from the biological sciences to characterize such phenomena. Thus, far from pertaining solely to the study of individual phenomena, the biological sciences also contribute to understanding human populations. As has become increasingly clear over the last several decades, health is a result of both social and biological determinants – and therefore, we need *both* social and biological sciences to understand public health.

This need for interdisciplinary integration is one of the reasons why, in defining public health, we prefer to use the concept of population rather than that of collectivity, which is found in such proposals as that of "collective health" in Brazil. The terms collectivity and community allude to a form of social organization. The term "population" is broader, because it includes both the social and biological dimensions of human groups.

This is also why, though some have argued against it, we still prefer the term "public health" instead of other terms such as "social medicine" or "sociomedicine" (Mercer, 1987). These terms are acceptable when studying only the social dimension of health but do not substitute for the concept of public health, which, as we have just argued, is broader (Roemer, 1993). Indeed, what defines the essence of the new public health is not the exclusive use of certain sciences over others. The biological reductionism of the past should not be replaced by sociological reductionism. Rather, we need an integration effort among scientific disciplines. This is precisely the conceptual opening that stems from defining public health by reference to its population level of analysis.

1.6 The Practice of Public Health

Public health is not only a field of inquiry, but also a space for professional practice. This dimension also requires conceptual clarification. As an arena for action, the modern conception of public health goes beyond simple dichotomies, such as personal versus environmental services, preventive versus curative activities and public versus private responsibilities. Instead of lending itself to these dichotomies, public health addresses the systematic efforts to identify health needs and organize comprehensive services with a well-defined population base. It thus encompasses the information required for characterizing the conditions of the population and the mobilization of resources necessary for responding to such conditions. In this sense, the essence of public health is **the health of the public**. Therefore, it includes "the organization of personnel and facilities to provide all health services required for the promotion of health, prevention of disease, diagnosis and treatment of illnesses and physical, social and vocational rehabilitation (Terris, 1985).

Public health encompasses the concept of medical care, but not in its technical and interpersonal aspects as applied to individuals in clinical situations, but rather in its organizational dimension as related to groups of providers and users. In addition, public health includes coordination of those actions that have an impact on the health of the population, although they go beyond health services strictly speaking. An important factor in the emergence of this broad perspective on the practice of public health has been the growing involvement of governments in financing and providing all types of health services. Indeed, any original limitation placed on the public sector to organize only environmental or preventive services has been invalidated practically worldwide, as the State has assumed a dominant role in the health system, including personal medical care. Indeed, the largest share of resources currently spent by the public sector in almost all countries is earmarked for personal curative services, whether provided by private contractors or salaried government personnel (Frenk and Donabedian, 1987).

Finally, although we have defined research and practice separately, both refer to the same universe, which delimits the space for integrating the two faces of public health. Thus, the efforts to generate knowledge about health and to act upon it can be categorized along different dimensions. A first dimension refers to specific populations, such as children, women, older adults, Indigenous people or migrants. A second dimension has to do with disease categories, such as infectious problems, non-communicable diseases, mental health challenges or injuries. Lastly, the areas of application may be focused on risk factors, such as environmental and occupational exposures, nutrition, risky behaviors like smoking or social deprivation.

Conceptions about the limits and contents of the universe of public health have varied throughout history. Likewise, the definitions that we have proposed for the two dimensions of public health result from a historical development in which different conceptual models of knowledge and action in this field have been taking shape. As the history of thought is not a mere progression of ideas, many of these models persist today. It is thus important to become familiar with them.

1.7 Conceptual Models in Public Health

Because the boundaries among fields of knowledge do not come from an intrinsic or predetermined division of reality, the first step in the development of a discipline or profession is "to construct the object" (Bourdieu et al., 1991). As noted above, the health field includes two major objects of analysis: conditions and responses. This distinction is useful for identifying the principal conceptual models that have guided public health, as depicted schematically in Table 1.2.

In simplified form, we suggest that conditions have historically been analyzed from two main perspectives: health and disease. The limits between the two are not always obvious; in fact, the most comprehensive conceptions go beyond this dichotomy.

Table 1.2 Conceptual models in public health. Adapted from Frenk (1993a)

Social response: objects of intervention	Conditions: analytical perspectives	
	Health	**Disease**
Individual/family	Hygienist/preventive model	Biomedical model
Biophysical environment	Sanitarist model	Classic epidemiological model
	Ecologist model	
Social environment	Sociomedical model	Social epidemiological model

However, public health thinking has included two main currents that, as Dubos reminds us, go back to the worship of Aesculapius, the Greek god of medicine, versus Hygieia, the Greek goddess of cleanliness (Dubos, 1959). One focuses on the study of disease; the other, while not excluding disease, seeks to understand the determinants of health in a broad conception that includes human development and well-being.

The social response to health and disease conditions may be directed to different objects of intervention. Historically, the main objects have been the individual, including their immediate family surroundings, and the environment, which can be subdivided into the biophysical and the social components. Crossing these two dimensions produces the typology of models shown in Table 1.2. The names given to the models correspond to the main historical currents of thinking about health. For example, the "hygienist/preventive" model was developed considerably in the nineteenth century, when there was a movement to instruct the family on a series of rules for behavior that defined a "healthy life," and came to constitute what Foucault has called "a morality of the body" (Foucault, 1973). This model was displaced by the "biomedical model," which brought the control of specific diseases to the center of public health concerns (Rosen, 1972), but eventually reappeared in programs aimed at changing individual behaviors and lifestyles as a basic strategy of health promotion (Frenk, 1979). Increasingly, we are seeing the emergence of a new model, through "One Health" or "planetary health" approaches, which seek to position not just humans, but also the environment, including animals, and Earth's natural resources as equal objects of analysis (Horton et al., 2014; Adisasmito et al., 2022).

Not all the conceptual models fit perfectly into the proposed categories. For example, the "ecologist model," whose principal exponent is Dubos (Dubos, 1959), seeks to transform both the physical and social environments. The "sociomedical model" encompasses very diverse conceptions whose single common denominator is that they all attempt to explain health phenomena in society. We will not undertake an exhaustive analysis of each of the models; our purpose has simply been to show the wealth of intellectual traditions that have characterized public health. Each of them has implied a particular program of development for acquisition of knowledge and for action in public health (Alvarado, 1976).

1.8 Public Health versus Population Health

In recent years, the term **population health** has emerged as an alternative to public health. Authors using this term often come from two separate traditions.

In the first tradition, population health has been used by social scientists to emphasize the role of broader determinants in health outcomes. Thus, social and economic factors are emphasized, in contrast to biological factors or clinical services. The consideration of population health as a distinct scientific approach grew out of work by Evans, Barer and Marmor in the 1990s (Coyte et al., 1995). Since then, researchers have proposed that the field be characterized by work focusing on health outcomes, patterns of health determinants and policies and interventions that link these patterns and outcomes (Kindig and Stoddart, 2003). This notion has further evolved into the assertion that population health as a field provides the scientific foundation for public health practice by providing the research results necessary to develop evidence-based interventions (Shultz et al., 2021). Such an interpretation suggests an important distinction between population health and public health. It claims that the field of population health, which here centers on the distribution of health conditions within a population, relies on public health to implement actionable responses to address population-level health concerns holistically. In other words, this tradition contrasts population health with public health, referring to population health as research and public health as practice.

In the second tradition, the term population health is increasingly used in medical education and by health care actors to define the role that medical professionals can play in improving the health of groups of people. For example, the American Medical Association defines population health as "improving the medical outcomes of people in a specific population" through health promotion, early screening and disease management (American Medical Association, 2023). In this definition, population health refers to the activities that health care professionals in a defined setting implement for a group of patients, by contrast with both individual clinical care and public health. Defining a specific population under the care of a group of providers can have implications for payment formulas based on the attainment of specific health outcomes in that population.

It is interesting to note that these two traditions are in direct opposition to each other, with the first one focusing on broader social determinants, while the second one focuses only on proximate medical outcomes within specific groups of people, at the exclusion of societal factors.

1.9 A Final Word on Definitions

The recent focus on the term population health underscores the risk of conceptual confusion that has complicated previous efforts to define public health. As mentioned at the start of this chapter, different actors have infused the term public health with distinct meanings, depending on their discipline, context and traditions. Our broad definition, for example, contrasts with the one proposed by the Centers for Diseases Control and Prevention in the United States (DeSalvo et al., 2017), which still defines public health in opposition to health care, therefore implying that the organization of personal health services is outside the scope of public health.

We will come back to these concepts when considering health systems in Chapter 7, and the distinction between personal and public health services, including what we call hybrid and population health services. Overall, we believe that these debates are a testament to the field's intrinsic complexity and multidisciplinarity. Ultimately, what truly matters is how specific definitions of the field favored by different societies guide which questions are asked, which answers are sought and which actions are taken.

1.10 Summary

In this chapter, we have seen the importance of laying out a conceptual framework for our understanding of public health. We have defined the term public health as the health conditions of populations and the social responses to these conditions: "public," as we use it, refers to populations; and by "health" we are concerning ourselves with both health conditions and responses to those conditions, devoid of any predefined value or goal attached to them. We have conceptualized public health as both an interdisciplinary field of inquiry and a space for professional practice (Mercer, 1987). We have also explored the intellectual evolution of the field, which has at times focused on the prevention or management of disease, and at others encompassed a broader concept of health to include human development and well-being. The conception of public health also evolved from a narrower view of the individual or family as the object of intervention, to a more comprehensive focus on the biophysical and social environment within which people live, including the Earth's natural systems. Finally, we have discussed how our proposed definition compares with alternative definitions of public health and population health in use currently.

Chapter 2 will apply a similar framework to the concept of global health, which is an extension of the scope of public health.

Comprehension and Discussion Questions

- This chapter proposes a broad conception of public health. In your experience, have you encountered a different definition of public health? If so, what was it and what are its strengths and weaknesses?
- Do you think a definition of public health should be neutral or explicitly consider values? What are the pros and cons of each approach?
- Consider the five different meanings of "public" presented at the start of the chapter. If we apply each of these to the concept of "public health," how does it change what you might study or the kind of work you might do in the field? What's your own definition of the word "public"?
- According to the chapter, what are the differences between the concepts of public health and medical care?
- Do you consider public health to be a discipline? Do you think it is important for public health to be interdisciplinary? Why?

Papers from Which This Chapter Is Adapted

Frenk, J. The new public health. *Annual Review of Public Health*, 1993, 14, 469–489.

Chapter 2 What Is Global Health?

Learning Objectives

- Describe how the concepts of international health and global health have evolved over the years.
- Identify a working definition of global health.
- Explain several ways in which globalization has increased the spread of health threats across borders, as well as health opportunities.
- Describe, differentiate and illustrate the concepts of interdependence and interconnection, and their relevance to public health in a globalized world.

2.1 Introduction

Global health has been rising on the global public agenda since at least the turn of the millennium. The COVID-19 pandemic has reinforced the recognition of global health as an issue that can touch all facets of political, economic and social life across all countries. Yet, despite its increasing importance, global health has developed in the absence of an academic tradition that can guide its efforts to generate knowledge and inform practice. As in the case of public health more broadly, it is necessary to develop a firm conceptual base for the concept of global health.

This is the focus of this chapter. In Chapter 1, we laid out a conceptual framework for public health. In this chapter, we now turn our attention to the global level. We explore and critique various working definitions of global health, explaining how they have been shaped by political and socioeconomic factors. We then propose our own definition of global health. Finally, we look at health conditions at the global level and the international transfer of health risks. Later, in Chapter 12, we will move to the organized social response at the global level and explain the concept of the global health system. Chapter 14 shows how this broader conception of global health can help analyze the response to a major public health crisis, such as the COVID-19 pandemic.

2.2 Defining Global Health

There are many working definitions of global health. Some emphasize certain types of health conditions (e.g., communicable diseases); whereas others center on certain populations of interest (e.g., people with lower incomes), focus on a certain group of countries (e.g., the Global South) or have a specific mission (e.g., equity). The scope and contents of the concept can profoundly influence what actors in the field research, finance, teach and/or do – in other words, how we think about global health shapes how we act on it

(Campbell et al., 2012). The concept of global health continues to evolve, and the range of possible definitions is wide. For example, Beaglehole and Bonita define global health as "collaborative trans-national research and action for promoting health for all," emphasizing a normative goal (Beaglehole and Bonita, 2010). Fried and colleagues (Fried, 2010, p. 535) argue that "global health and public health are indistinguishable," that the concepts are basically the same, since they both focus on the population level of analysis even if global health refers to the entire world (Fried et al., 2010). And King and Koski (2020, p.1) argue that global health is "public health somewhere else," calling on practitioners to examine their assumptions of why one would practice public health "somewhere else." The boundaries of the concept may also be expanding. "One Health" is the concept that the health of humans, animals and the environment are inextricably intertwined, and should be understood and acted upon accordingly (World Health Organization, 2017). "Planetary health" extends even further, linking human health to that of the planet in light of the profound health implications of climate change and environmental degradation more broadly (Horton et al., 2014).

Global health encompasses many dimensions, but each of them in isolation offers only a partial perspective. In our view, global health should be defined by two key elements: its level of analysis, which involves the entire population of the world; and the relationships of interdependence that bind together the units of social organization making up the global population (e.g., nation states, private organizations, civil society movements and others). The focus is indeed on human health, while recognizing that determinants of human health reach far and wide, including to the planetary level.

The term "global health" began to replace "international health" in the 2000s, and the two concepts should be distinguished from each other. Since it was coined, around the creation of the International Health Commission in 1913 by the Rockefeller Foundation (Brown et al., 2006), the term international health has been identified with the control of epidemics across borders and with the health needs of low-income and middle-income countries (Godue, 1992). Various textbooks and training programs also included in this term the health of Indigenous people of high-income countries. Supporters of this view regarded international needs as alien and peripheral, and very frequently as threats. Consistent with these ideas, international activities were identified as aid and defense and were delivered through unilateral perspectives. The international health agenda was also affected by the idea that most health needs could be fully addressed with technology (Gómez-Dantés, 2001). This notion is still prevalent among various global health initiatives (Birn, 2005; Samb et al., 2009). "The temptation to pin all hope on the latest technology remains every bit as powerful as it was in the near past," said Judith Rodin in 2007, then president of the Rockefeller Foundation (Rodin, 2007). This reductionist perspective contrasts with the growing realization that most global health problems have strong behavioral, cultural, social, political and economic determinants that demand comprehensive – not only technical – approaches.

International health also placed excessive emphasis on "vertical" programs devoted to control specific diseases such as smallpox or malaria and paid little attention to health systems as a whole, with well-documented consequences such as islands of well-resourced programs within weaker health systems (Samb et al., 2009). The shortcomings of vertical approaches have repeatedly prompted calls for a shift to a "horizontal" focus on health systems, such as primary health care or universal health coverage. Jaime Sepúlveda argued for a "diagonal" perspective that would use explicit intervention priorities to drive improvements into the health system (Sepúlveda, 2006). Nevertheless, debates and tensions between vertical and horizontal approaches remain a perennial feature of the global health landscape.

International health cooperation has traditionally fallen under the rubric of foreign aid – support for polio eradication and treatment of HIV/AIDS are prominent examples. But the very concept of aid conveys an asymmetric image in which problems and risks flow from the Global South to the Global North, whereas resources and solutions move in the opposite direction. This view fails to capture the reality of health interdependence. It also fails to consider major shifts in the global distribution of resources, influence, capabilities and needs as emerging powers continue their expansion.

A sort of linguistic modernization has revitalized the traditional contents attributed to international health through the use and dissemination of the notion of global health. In the media, in lay and scientific literature and in major initiatives, global health has been identified with problems supposedly characteristic of developing countries, and global cooperation in health with a sort of paternalistic philanthropy that is armed with the technological developments of the advanced industrialized countries. Unfortunately, it is again the stereotypical idea of the poor, ignorant, passive and traditional societies in need of the charity and technology of the rich that prevails in the use of this term.

More recently, a growing movement has called to "decolonize" global health, arguing that its governance structure and practice is a direct legacy of the colonial era (Abimbola et al., 2021). These calls can be understood as a reaction and critique of the aforementioned conceptualization, underscoring the importance of redefining the term itself. Critics argue that more attention should be paid to power imbalances in the funding and implementation of global health programs, the leadership of global health organizations and the production of knowledge itself through research. A watershed moment was the COVID-19 pandemic, when inequities in access to vaccines highlighted the shortcomings of the current system. More generally, this movement reflects a moment of geopolitical realignment, with many countries in the Global South being increasingly critical of a Western-dominated international system.

In a sense, global health, as it is understood and practiced today, fails to capture the essence of globalization, much like its predecessor notion of international health. In a real sense, we need to reimagine and globalize the concept of global health.

To this end, we propose to move beyond reductionist definitions and to reconceptualize global health to reflect two key notions. First, global health should not be viewed as "foreign health," but rather as the health of the global population. Second, global health should be understood not as a manifestation of dependence, but rather as the product of health interdependence, a process that has arisen in parallel with economic, environmental and geopolitical interdependence (Chen et al., 1996).

The core idea behind the notion of health interdependence is that no stakeholder – not even the most powerful government or corporation – is singlehandedly able to address all the health threats that affect it. The COVID-19 pandemic illustrated just how profoundly interdependent the world is. Many determinants of health – such as the dissemination of patterns of work, lifestyles, diets and other aspects of consumption – that are conducive to diseases once thought to affect only rich societies – diabetes, cardiovascular disease, cancer – have become globalized and are now affecting many of the world's poorer citizens in equal or greater measure.

Table 2.1 Health in populations: two essential dimensions. Based on Frenk and Moon (2013)

Dimension	National level	Global level
Health conditions	National epidemiological profile	Global transfer of health risks
Organized social response	National health system	Global health systems

Like public health, global health is defined by the population level of analysis – in this case, the entire world population. This means that the same framework we used in the first chapter can be applied now. As discussed then, when thinking about health in populations, we must analyze two essential dimensions: health conditions (e.g., diseases and risk factors) and the way in which a society responds to those conditions. This framework can be applied at both the national level and the global level, as shown in Table 2.1. Faced with a set of health conditions, a country responds through its national health system. At the global level, the key concept in understanding the pattern of health conditions is the "international transfer of health risks" – that is, the way in which the movement of people, products, resources and lifestyles across borders can contribute to the spread of disease (Frenk et al., 1997). Globalization has intensified cross-border health threats (Keohane and Nye, 2001), leading to a situation of health interdependence – the notion that no nation or organization is able to address singlehandedly the health threats it faces but instead must rely to some degree on others to mount an effective response (Frenk et al., 1997). The organized social response to health conditions at the global level is what we call the "global health system," and the way in which the system is managed is what we refer to as "governance."

2.3 Global Transfer of Health Threats and Opportunities

Although communicable diseases such as pandemic influenza, malaria or HIV/AIDS have attracted the greatest amount of international health funding, political attention and institutional innovation (Institute for Health Metrics and Evaluation, 2012), what were once regarded as problems only of low-income countries, such as many common infections, malnutrition and maternal deaths, are no longer the only problems of such countries. Low-income countries also carry the heaviest burden of many non-communicable diseases, mental disorders and injuries. In health terms, for nearly two decades, high- and middle-income countries have been more alike than different (Bloom, 2005; Ferrari et al., 2024). Non-communicable diseases have attracted increased political attention, as their growing burden adds to and sometimes outweighs that of communicable diseases in many low-income and middle-income countries (Vos et al., 2020).

At the same time, the COVID-19 pandemic made clear that communicable diseases will remain a threat in high-income countries, and that wealth alone does not determine how well a society can manage such threats. For example, measles outbreaks have resurged in the United States and Europe due to growing numbers of parents being unwilling to vaccinate their children, among other barriers to immunization (Wilder-Smith and Qureshi, 2020). Threats such as the spread of antimicrobial resistance and the risks of (re-)emerging infectious diseases linked to environmental degradation and urbanization remain major challenges for higher-income countries and lower-income countries alike.

The traditional binary classification of communicable and non-communicable diseases fails to capture an additional type of health determinant, which generates a novel category of health challenges – those arising directly from globalization. Irrespective of the type of resulting disease, global health risks spread through common processes created to support production, communication, trade and travel worldwide (Lee et al., 2009b). These risks do not necessarily move from the Global South to North. For example, an often-overlooked example of the transfer of health risks is the establishment of polluting factories in developing nations, transplanted from industrialized countries to take advantage of weaker regulatory environments. Indeed, all countries, irrespective of their location, wealth, history or culture, are exposed to common health threats associated with globalization. At the same time, the increased interdependence produced by globalization can generate new benefits and opportunities; every country can benefit from ideas, knowledge, goods, regulatory approaches and skills originating elsewhere (Frenk et al., 1997).

Although the links between globalization and health are complex (Huynen et al., 2005), the transfer of health risks and opportunities can be organized into six broad categories, as shown in Table 2.2: cross-border movement of elements of the natural environment; people; production of goods and services (e.g., global value chains in manufacturing); consumption of goods and services (e.g., food, tobacco, narcotics, health care); information, knowledge and culture; and rules (Frenk et al., 1997).

These six types of flows underscore the conclusion that no country – whether high, low, or middle income – can be isolated from the risks that emerge elsewhere. Such interconnections are not necessarily new, but the intensification of cross-border trade, travel and communication that are the hallmarks of globalization have strengthened them and, in many cases, have created situations not merely of interconnection, but also of interdependence. Indeed, perhaps the two most striking features of global health today are interconnectedness – both across countries and across sectors – in the causes and effects of health threats, and interdependence in our capacity to respond to them effectively.

It is important to distinguish between interconnection and interdependence. Interconnection describes the nature of health threats and effects, whereas interdependence refers to the distribution of power, responsibility and capacity to respond. For the very powerful, such as governments of large wealthy countries, some health threats may be interconnected across borders but do not automatically imply interdependence, since these countries can manage some of these specific threats alone (Fidler, 2011). However, for many others, particularly smaller, less wealthy countries, or communities that live in closer proximity to neighboring countries, interdependence is a defining feature of the domestic health landscape. Examples of health challenges linked to interdependence include regulation of the quality of imported food, medicines, manufactured goods and inputs; getting timely access to information about the global spread of infectious diseases; procurement of sufficient vaccine and drug supplies in a pandemic; and ensuring a sufficient corps of well-trained health personnel in the face of migration ("brain drain").

Table 2.2 Cross-border flows that generate threats and opportunities of globalization for health. Adapted from Frenk et al. (2014)

	Examples of threats	Examples of opportunities
Elements of the natural environment	Environmental threats (e.g., climate change, air and water pollution); spread of pathogens (e.g., animal-borne illnesses such as avian influenza)	Improved access to natural resources (e.g., water)
People	Spread of pathogens (e.g., human-to-human transmission)	Spread of knowledge and skills through workforce movement
Production of goods and services	Transplantation of harmful practices (e.g., high-polluting factories to countries with weaker regulatory systems); changing labor conditions enabling adoption of sedentary lifestyles that contribute to metabolic disorders	Economic growth and technology transfer
Consumption of goods and services	Spread of harmful products (e.g., tobacco); global trade in unhealthy foods	Spread of useful medical technologies; adoption of health-enhancing goods and services
Information, knowledge and culture	Inappropriate use of technologies (e.g., leading to antimicrobial resistance); spread of misinformation (e.g. anti-vaccination content on social media)	Spread of health-related knowledge and practices that enhance health and well-being, such as family planning; cross-fertilization and access to new knowledge, whether traditional or modern
Rules	Trans-national investment treaties restricting national regulatory policies; trans-national intellectual property rules increasing drug prices	Health-focused trans-national rules, such as the WHO Framework Convention on Tobacco Control, expanding national policy space for health protection

Additionally, these challenges are interconnected across sectors – that is, their causes and the management of their effects do not sit neatly within the traditional boundaries of the health sector or within the sole control of health officials. Rather, an intricate web of governmental and non-governmental players (e.g., private firms, civil society organizations, the media and academic institutions) all exercise some measure of influence over these health threats and the collective responses to them. Situations of complex interdependence frequently result, with many players working across different scales and sectors ultimately shaping health outcomes.

An example of a health threat due to the production of a good (gasoline) spread across borders, and how an opportunity to address that threat also arose because of the spread of knowledge, ideas, goods (technologies) and rules across borders is given in Box 2.1.

Box 2.1 Unleaded gasoline, a global health issue at your local petrol station

The year 2021, when Algeria's service stations stopped offering it, officially marked the end of leaded petrol worldwide (United Nations Environment Programme, 2021). This was the final act of a public health and environment catastrophe that started in 1922, when tetraethyl lead was first added to petrol to improve engine performance. Soon, scientists linked it to stroke, cancer and brain damage, especially in small children.

Gasoline may seem like a national, if not local affair, but it is a perfect example of the interconnection and interdependence concepts described in this chapter. Leaded gasoline was first developed by General Motors in the United States. By the 1970s, the majority of petrol produced around the world contained lead, showing how fast harmful products and goods can be disseminated. Similarly, while most high-income countries prohibited the use of leaded petrol in the 1980s, it took a concerted international effort, including scientists, public health advocates and policy-makers, another four decades to eliminate leaded petrol across the world. The widespread diffusion of scientific evidence, alongside regulatory policies and technological transfer to upgrade oil refineries, all played a role in this success story.

2.4 Summary

Global health challenges are not only the diseases of the world's poorest communities, but rather comprise all components of the triple burden of disease: first, the unfinished agenda of infections, malnutrition and reproductive health problems; second, the emerging challenges represented by non-communicable diseases, mental disorders and injuries; and third, the health risks directly associated with globalization. Globalization has intensified both health threats and opportunities that cross borders, increasing interconnection across countries. It has also increased interdependence among countries in managing these threats and opportunities. Global health challenges include all issues beyond any one country's capacity to address, and often require concerted responses from governments and non-State actors.

Next, we turn our attention to the question of how we define health and how we can quantify it.

Comprehension and Discussion Questions

- Consider the discussion of the concept of public health in Chapter 1, and the concept of global health presented in this chapter. What are the key similarities between these two concepts? What are some key differences?
- The term "global health" marks a shift from the previous widely used term, "international health." What are key differences between these two terms, and what might have led to the change in terminology?
- What is the difference between interconnection and interdependence? Provide examples of these two concepts for a health topic in which you are interested.
- How has the COVID-19 pandemic influenced your understanding of the concept of global health?

Papers from Which This Chapter is Adapted

Frenk, J., Gomez-Dantes, O. & Moon, S. 2014. From sovereignty to solidarity: a renewed concept of global health for an era of complex interdependence. *The Lancet*, 383, 94–97.

Section

2

Health: Definitions, Domains and Determinants

Chapter 3 Health Conditions

Learning Objectives

- Understand different definitions of health and the way in which the definition influences the scope of issues addressed by public health research and action.
- Define and distinguish between the concepts of health conditions, health needs and health priorities.
- Explore what shapes those concepts and how they may evolve over time or place.
- Relate the concept of health needs to the medical care process and the relationship between patient and provider.

3.1 Introduction

As the German nineteenth-century philosopher Arthur Schopenhauer famously said, "Health is not everything, but without health there is nothing." In this chapter, we will deepen our definition of "health," and what determines it. Health, the foundational object of our field, is intrinsically complex, and ours is probably the profession that has the biggest problem defining the object that distinguishes it. This seemingly simple definition has been the subject of some of the most enduring debates in our field.

We also live in an era of medicalization, where more and more domains of life fall under the heading of health. Nutrition, for example, is now considered to be an aspect of health – so much so that schools of public health have departments of nutrition. Parenting is considered a health issue, as is aging. This medicalization of life has huge implications on where we set the limits of the health system. Without clarity on what health is, the boundaries of the health system become permeable – and that is exactly what has happened. If someone is slightly unhappy, should they be treated medically? In many places they are. What about if they have a high risk for disease but do not yet meet the criteria for illness? There are no right answers here, but this is more than an intellectual exercise. The definitions we use have practical implications for how we set priorities for health.

3.2 What Is Health?

The dawn of a new era in the evolution of human health was emblematically encapsulated in the now classical definition that is part of the preamble of the World Health Organization's (WHO) constitution. Carefully drafted in 1946, it defines health as (World Health Organization, 1946):

> A state of complete physical, mental, and social well-being and not merely the absence of disease or infirmity.

Since those heroic days, there have been several attempts to adapt this definition to the circumstances of the twenty-first century. New conceptual developments and a changing context are demanding the design of a definition better suited to the increasing complexity of global health. The evolution of global health can be illustrated by various elements, including a transition in the health conditions of the global population (epidemiological transition) – most notably the rise of chronic diseases and the emergence of new infectious diseases – and a transition in the response to those conditions (health care transition) (Lerner, 1973; Caldwell J, 1990; Frenk et al., 1991a; McCracken and Phillips, 2017). Critics of the WHO characterization stress the need for a "dynamic definition," a "more specific or narrow definition," a "practical definition" and even a "less tyrannical definition" (Dolfman, 1973; Fitzgerald, 1994; Saracci, 1997; Bircher, 2005).

We respect the fact that the WHO's definition was aspirational, and a very advanced conceptualization for its time. However, we have a number of concerns about it. First, the use of the term "state" is problematic. It tends to convey the idea of permanency or immovability. It is a static notion. Those that criticize the use of this term tend to view health more as a "process" or a dynamic condition, implying continuous adjustments to the changing demands of the physical and social environment (Dubos, 1965).

A second important objection to the WHO definition is its use of the term "complete" when referring to well-being. There are multiple states of health that are less than completely perfect health. The requirement for complete health "would leave most of us unhealthy most of the time," says Richard Smith, former editor of the *BMJ* (Smith, 2008). At a time when chronic illness increasingly dominates the epidemiological landscape, the emphasis on total or absolute "physical, mental and social well-being" seems unrealistic. In his paper "Ecological observations of the relation of physical illness, mental illness, and social environment," Hinkle (1961) states:

> Even the "most healthy" people in our society nearly always have dental caries, sometimes have colds, sometimes have accidents, sometimes become anxious or depressed, [and] not infrequently experience an elevated blood pressure or become obese.

Healthy people, he concludes, are not disease-free, they simply have less disease than unhealthy people.

An associated problem with the institutional endorsement of a "perfect state of wellness" is the possibility of confusing an aspiration with a norm, which in this case implies accepting the idea that physical, mental and social well-being is not only desirable and attainable but also expected. When such an endorsement is backed by the coercive power of the State, it can lead to concepts of "normalcy" and "deviance" that are susceptible to human rights violations against members of a society who do not conform to the expected norm. In the former Soviet Union, for example, political dissidents were diagnosed as social deviants for not conforming to certain norms (Bloch and Reddaway, 1977). Is someone socially unwell and in need of medical treatment if they object to the way the government is functioning? Whoever defines what conformity to social norms and expectations entails can have a lot of influence under this definition – too much influence, we would argue. This idea of social well-being leads to a slippery slope that equates health with conformity to social expectations.

Some have extended this definition further to include not only the well-being of the individual but also "the social, emotional, spiritual and cultural well-being of the whole community" (National Health and Medical Research Council, 1996). This extended goal is not as widely accepted as one might think. Some authors believe that these definitions equate health with happiness, spiritual fulfillment and social content, and considerably broaden the health care horizon to include character flaws, existential anguish, spiritual doubt, aging, poverty and crime, all of which are considered sickness or, at least, problems amenable to medical treatment (Steinfels, 1973). Most of these authors have argued that health, happiness and social content refer to distinct life experiences. Saracci, for example, states that "common existential problems – involving emotions, passions, personal values, and questions on the meaning of life – can make your days less than happy or even frankly uncomfortable, but they are not reducible to health problems" (Saracci, 1997, p. 1409).

Transforming all sorts of personal and social complaints into health conditions and turning them over to health care providers is not only conceptually incorrect, but it also has the additional disadvantage of reducing personal autonomy and placing too much power and authority in the hands of the medical profession. "In particular, given our training and expertise," says Fitzgerald, "we healthcare professionals are no more competent to treat social distress than other citizens" (Fitzgerald, 1994).

In opposition to the more expansive views, Callahan proposes to define health simply as "a state of physical well-being," and adds (Callahan, 1973):

> That state need not be "complete," but it must be at least adequate, i.e., without significant impairment of function. It also need not encompass "mental" well-being; one can be healthy yet anxious, well yet depressed. And it surely ought not to encompass "social well-being," except insofar as that well-being will be impaired by the presence of large-scale, serious physical infirmities.

Given the biological basis of many mental disorders and the important progress that has been made in their medical treatment, it would be difficult to generate a consensus around a definition of health that omits "mental well-being." Certainly, we do not mean to suggest that mental health problems should not be the purview of medicine. The value of Callahan's proposal, however, is that it points to the need for a definition of health that is specific and operational, while circumscribing the participation of health care professionals only to those domains of life where the positive contribution of medicine has been clearly demonstrated.

We also question the WHO's use of the adverb "merely," because it does not invite a reflection on what else is lacking and it blurs the temporal dimension. When we talk about absence of disease, are we talking about both present states of health and future health? If someone falls down dead later today, were they healthy in the morning? Is the "mere" absence of disease related to their future state? Saying health is not the absence of disease does not help us understand exactly what it is.

3.3 Health Conditions versus Needs

We must also make clear the distinction between "health conditions" and "health needs." Health needs are a subset of health conditions: they are those conditions that require care. It is crucial for us to use these terms precisely not to satisfy some idiosyncratic preference, but because these definitions have implications for policy, for how we address health in our community.

To explain what we believe is a good working definition of health conditions, we need to first introduce a short list of attributes that will form the basis for that definition:

Multidimensional: Health conditions occur in a broad set of situations and affect people and society on many levels. They are more than just diseases.

Objective and subjective: They include aspects that someone else can observe and measure, such as an echocardiogram of the heart, as well as those that are perceived by the individual. An accountant may have a different sense of health upon losing a finger than a violinist would.

Present and future: These processes have a temporal aspect. I might feel perfectly healthy in the morning and drop dead of a heart attack in the afternoon. Clearly, I was not as healthy in the morning as I seemed.

External and internal: Health conditions involve both the internal structures and functions of the body and the person's adaptability to their physical and social environment.

So, our definition describes health conditions as a multidimensional set of situations, with both subjective and objective measures, related to present and future structures and functions of the human body, as well as the capacity to adapt to both the physical and social environment in which human beings live.

3.4 Intensity Gradient

Health, as we've already noted, is not just one static state (Donabedian, 1973). There is an intensity gradient to health, a range between this ideal of perfect health and the complete absence of health, which is death. The distinctions we make below are not perfect – even death has a gradient today, because there is a difference between being brain dead, when your organs might still be available for donation, and being dead beyond the reach of medicine. But they give us a starting point for understanding the concept of gradients.

As Figure 3.1 shows, there is a range from extreme health to extreme loss of health. (As public health professionals, when we talk about the end of life, we refer to the *death*

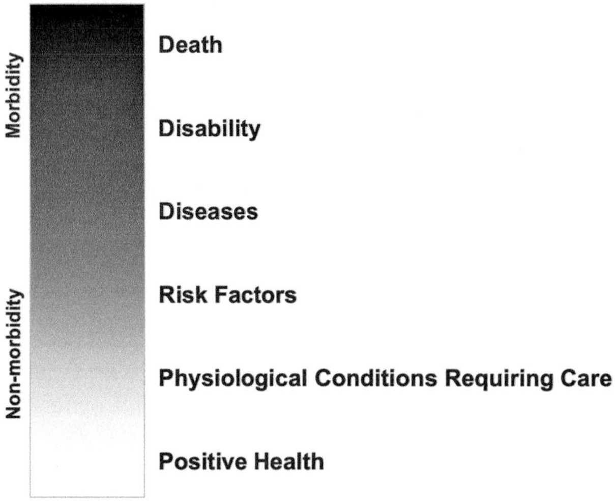

Figure 3.1 Health conditions: the intensity gradient.

of an individual and the *mortality* rate of a population.) We can be alive, but have different degrees of disability, such as needing a wheelchair or being blind. We can have specific diseases. Risk factors can include behaviors like smoking, which boosts the risk of disease, but is not in and of itself a disease, unless you consider it an addiction. Physiological conditions that require care include pregnancy, which is obviously essential for the survival and maintenance of our species, and the growth and development of young children. These are health conditions, because if they are not taken care of they can lead to disability and death, but they are not in and of themselves "unhealthy." Positive health can be defined, as Donabedian does, as having a functional reserve. This includes the concept of resilience, the capacity to respond under conditions of stress, and the ability to adapt to changing environments. The distinctions between states of health as described above are also somewhat arbitrary. The development and growth of children, for example, is an indicator of good health. But it is nevertheless a condition that requires care. The capacity to get pregnant, for example, is not per se an indicator of good or bad health. But the event called pregnancy becomes a condition that requires care.

3.5 Health Needs

In sum, a health need is a condition that requires care. The word "need" is often used to refer to health services: "I need to see a doctor right now." Or to resources: "This community needs a hospital." But we are reserving the use of the word need for health conditions. Except for hypochondriacs, seeing a doctor is a means to an end, not a need in and of itself. The end is to improve a health condition. These are not just semantic distinctions. A need is a situation that if not addressed may produce a negative consequence, either at the individual or at the population level. For example, during the COVID-19 pandemic, asymptomatic patients may not have been considered as having conditions that required care. After all, if they did not experience any negative consequence themselves, was there a need? It is the knowledge that they could infect more vulnerable individuals that led us to consider their conditions a health need. This is a deeply conceptual point because it means that we do not lose our focus on the real need that we are trying to address. Everything else – medications, facilities, human resources, technology – are means to that end.

Let us consider some key points regarding health needs. As we have already stated, health needs are a subset of health conditions. Furthermore, the concept of health needs is a social construction. The same behavior can be interpreted as a health need in one social condition but not another. A murder can be a crime or an expression of mental illness – not guilty by reason of insanity. Historically, many diseases, such as leprosy, were considered divine punishment, not a health condition. Even in the early days of the HIV/AIDS epidemic some viewed the disease as punishment for homosexual activities. There are also some diseases today, such as chronic fatigue syndrome, for which we do not have a good medical response. At the opposite end of the spectrum, we have conditions that historically were not considered health needs, but are now, because of medicalization. Drug addiction, for instance, can be seen as a crime and a moral failing, or – as we prefer to view it – as a health need. Medicalization is not always a bad thing; sometimes it can be the most enlightened response. But it is a value judgment, so this notion of need is always a social construct.

Another point that is important here is that different groups in society have different definitions of health needs. What a doctor sees as a health need may not be what patients see as health needs and vice versa. As Donabedian explains, a lot of what we consider unmet needs arise because we do not agree on what is needed (Donabedian, 1973). Preventive or early detection services might be considered essential by the medical profession, for example. The medical profession believes every child needs health services in the form of vaccines to be healthy. Some parents, on the other hand, take a different perspective, declining vaccines out of a concern regarding the relative risk of harm. The opposite is also true: there are conditions that people might feel require care and the profession might consider illegitimate. Several conditions, like chronic fatigue and fibromyalgia, have gone through periods where sufferers considered their problem to be medical, but the profession did not. Alternative therapies, like chiropractic services, might be another example where the general public may consider them a medical treatment, but health regulators may not, because there is no science to support their use. (Of course, much of what we do in Western medicine also lacks scientific support, but that is a topic for a different discussion.) Problems can also arise when the profession acts as an arm of the State, as cited above with the Soviet Union and mental health. This potential inconsistency between the professional definition of needs and the popular definition of needs is a pervasive problem in the health system, particularly in prevention and health promotion.

It is also important to make a clear distinction between what we mean by disease, illness and sickness. These terms are often used interchangeably, but their differences are crucial. Diseases can be diagnosed and treated. An illness is the way a person experiences disease. And sickness refers to the social role that people who are sick can play. Those who are sick are allowed to stay home from work or school. Sickness is a social role that people who have been diagnosed with a disease or who experience the illness are allowed socially to assume.

So, we see that there is a link between health conditions and response. The first element of the social response is to find which subset of conditions require care. This leads to identifying the substantive areas of public health. If we start with the presence of reasonably objective measurable *conditions*, then – both through scientific evidence and social preferences – we define a subset of these as health *needs*. Donabedian's significant insight was to show that the process of determining health needs occurs in the context of information, research and policies. The first step of the social response to health conditions is to define health needs.

We consider the increasing problem of obesity in Box 3.1. In this example, obesity is widely considered a health condition, but there is disagreement on whether it is a health need or a health priority.

3.5.1 Health Priorities

As we have seen, it is important to understand which health conditions become needs so that we can then decide which needs to make a priority. Not all conditions and needs are a priority. There may be a health need for which there exists no effective treatment; Alzheimer's disease, the most common type of dementia, currently fits this category. The lack of a viable treatment to stop or slow Alzheimer's disease means society should invest in more research in this area. Similarly, there may exist a reasonably effective approach to a disease, but a lack of resources to pay for it, or the costs are so high that they prohibit

Box 3.1 Obesity: health need, health condition or health priority?

More than one billion people in the world now live with obesity, according to a 2024 *Lancet* study. Obesity among children and adolescents has quadrupled since the 1990s (Phelps et al., 2024). All public health actors agree there is a pressing need to better prevent, control and address this growing public health challenge. But one thing they disagree on is how to define obesity. In 2013, the American Medical Association officially recognized obesity as a disease. The WHO similarly defines obesity as a "chronic complex disease defined by excessive fat deposits that can impair health" (World Health Organization, 2024). Others disagree: the United Kingdom and Denmark, for example, do not consider obesity a disease but a risk factor (Vallgårda et al., 2017; Luli et al., 2023).

This debate is driven in part by difficulties in measuring obesity. The most used metric, the body mass index (BMI), is an outdated and imprecise measure for diagnosis because it does not take into account individual health markers and body fat distribution. For example, some thinner people can still be at increased risk for cardiovascular and metabolic complications because of the way they store fat. Decisions on how to classify obesity also reflect different contexts: the 2013 American Medical Association statement, for example, was in part an attempt to give the condition more legitimacy and increase access to health care. Finally, definitions proposed by the medical profession are also challenged by social movements to promote acceptance and eliminate social stigma around obesity.

This ongoing debate is not just semantic. How we define obesity has very real social, psychological and economic implications, more so since a new wave of effective but expensive weight-loss medications that target areas of the brain to regulate appetite entered the market in 2021. Who should be able to access those new drugs, especially in situations of scarcity or when high prices strain health budgets, is open for debate.

society from making this treatment a priority (Kremer, 2004). In this case, new or cheaper technology or pricing structures might be required. When HIV/AIDS medications first became available in the mid-1990s, for example, the combination therapies were quickly adopted in wealthy countries like the United States and most of Europe, but they were prohibitively expensive in low-income and middle-income countries. It took a dramatic reduction in prices to make these medications available in sub-Saharan Africa, which then made it possible for delivering these therapies to patients to become a top global priority. The COVID-19 pandemic further illustrates this distinction between health conditions and health priorities. The huge differences observed in terms of countries' responses to the pandemic, even among countries with similar levels of infection, reflected different prioritization processes, dependent in part on funding, treatment availability, perceived risk compared to other health threats or political conditions fostering disinformation.

3.6 The Medical Care Process and Environment

It is useful to break down the process of providing medical care into its constituent parts to gain deeper knowledge of health needs.

3.6.1 Patient and Provider Roles

As Donabedian explains in his 1973 classic, "The assessment of need," the provider and patient play different roles in the medical care process (Donabedian, 1973). Donabedian describes two parallel and related chains of activities and events arising in response to a need (Figure 3.2). Generally, the chain is started by a patient who perceives a medical need, say for a sinus infection, and goes to the provider for care. Sometimes the patient is directed to a provider by family members or others concerned about their condition. Once contact between the two occurs, the provider then tries to diagnose the need and decides how to address it, though of course the patient is also involved in the diagnostic process and must generally play some role, for instance, by taking medication, making different lifestyle choices or visiting other specialists or caregivers.

The point at which the patient uses the medical service is where the parallel chains converge and hopefully lead to a resolution of the need. The provider and patient often decide together when the need has been adequately addressed, though the patient can certainly make that decision unilaterally, as can the provider, though less often. Faced with a patient who has an apparent sinus infection, for instance, a doctor might decide either to prescribe an antibiotic or that the risk of promoting antibiotic resistance outweighs the modest benefit the patient will receive from the drug. Sometimes, of course, the need is not adequately addressed, because of an incorrect diagnosis or treatment.

As should be clear by now, this whole process takes place within a larger context. Before we worried about global antibiotic resistance, the patient with sinus pain would certainly have been prescribed an antibiotic, for instance; in some cases, doctors still do, because they want to be seen as doing something for their patient. In the United States, sometimes fear of lawsuits leads to an excess of care – such as brain scans for repeated

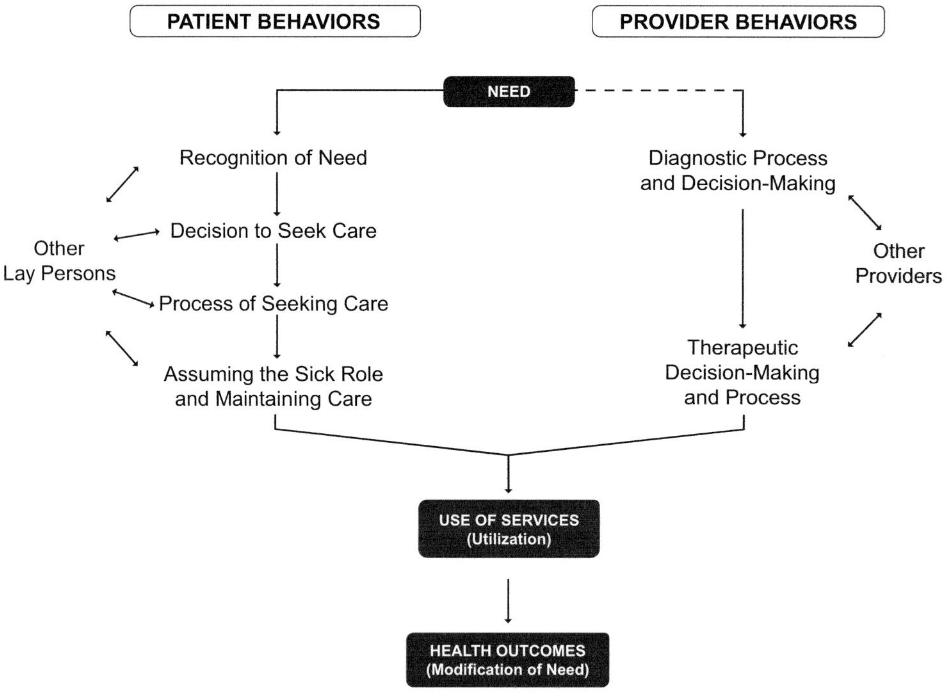

Figure 3.2 A model of the medical care process. Based on Donabedian, A., *Aspects of Medical Care Administration: Specifying Requirements for Health Care*. Cambridge, MA: Harvard University Press, 1973, pp. 58–88.

sinus headaches, to ensure there is no tumor. Similarly, decisions related to COVID-19 may have reflected a change in our understanding of disease patterns, through predictive modeling of cases and deaths, rather than a change in the patient's need itself. In all these cases, the social context influences the care the patient receives.

Medical care also has its own structures and processes, as anyone who has visited a doctor's office will understand. In the United States, Switzerland and many other countries where private insurance plays a major role in the health care system, the demands of insurance providers add another administrative layer. Governmental agencies and insurance companies in the United States, for instance, have the authority to decide which treatments are appropriate for many conditions and which will be reimbursed. In addition, these structures are overlaid with cultural and societal ones, which can influence need as well as responses to needs.

3.6.2 Patient and Provider Needs

Medical need is sometimes in the eye of the beholder. Not every medical need perceived by a patient will be seen the same way by the provider. A patient might worry that chest pains are a sign of a heart attack, while the provider is convinced that they are merely indigestion caused by overeating and no treatment is necessary. A provider who can find nothing wrong with a patient may decide that there is no cause for concern, while the patient's own experience suggests a different conclusion. Conversely, providers may believe their patients require cholesterol-lowering drugs, but because the patient does not perceive that need, the prescribed drugs never get taken.

These perceived needs can also change with time. Fifty years ago, if parents asked their provider for advice about a child who did not speak, did not make eye contact and rocked back and forth repeatedly, they might have been told that their child's condition was beyond medical help; the child should be institutionalized. Today, doctors, therapists and parents would aggressively treat such a child as early as possible in hopes of mitigating autism spectrum disorder symptoms. Similarly, many providers used to dismiss conditions such as fibromyalgia and chronic fatigue syndrome as psychosomatic – or "just in their patients' heads"– while today we take them more seriously as medical conditions. The increasing evidence supporting long COVID-19 followed a similar process: initially dubbed as a psychological issue, it is now increasingly recognized as a significant outcome of the infection.

Patients may also be suspicious of medical care because they are focused on their subjective experience, rather than on the science that (hopefully) undergirds the treatment. So, a patient who feels no better and maybe a little worse on a statin drug might stop taking the drug or decide after a few weeks that they have taken it long enough; while their provider would want them to continue the drug indefinitely in hopes of preventing future problems. Similarly, parents may distrust vaccines because they see their children scream in pain from the shot and have never lived through measles or whooping cough themselves; while providers, who have studied those diseases and the need for herd protection (when a disease can no longer spread through a population because of high levels of immunity), have an easier time looking past the child's cries.

Providers and patients may be particularly likely to have different views of medical needs if they come from different backgrounds, face different challenges and struggle in other aspects of their lives – especially if the provider does not make an effort to understand these contextual differences. This may be one explanation for the disparities of care that we see in the United States, for instance, particularly between White and African American, low-income communities (Mitchell and Perry, 2020). Patients whose providers are of a different race, wealth level or educational background may have more difficulty trusting their medical recommendations (Street et al., 2008).

As a society, we are generally more likely to accept the provider's views of needs – to see the doctor as the authority. At other times, public pressure or support for patients can change the medical establishment's outlook.

3.7 Summary

In sum, it is important to think critically about the definition of health. The (re) definition of this term should be a continuous endeavor. It requires the participation of various actors, including patients. It demands taking into account multiple cultural perspectives. And it should consider new knowledge and technological progress. Given the complex and dynamic nature of health, this process cannot aim at generating a once-and-for-all agreement on its precise meaning. Instead, it should provide a general framework that could guide further explorations to identify and measure the complex components and determinants of that elusive aspiration we call health.

Furthermore, it is important to understand the concept of health conditions, which are a multidimensional set of situations, with both subjective and objective measures, related to present and future structures and functions of the human body, as well as the capacity to adapt to both the physical and social environment in which human beings live. Health conditions occur on a gradient from an idealized state of perfect health to the total absence of health, which is death. Health needs are a subset of health conditions – they are the health conditions that require care.

The definition of health needs happens within a biological, social and political context. Health needs are a social construct and are likely to be perceived differently by different groups in society, such as health care providers and patients. Health priorities are a subset of health needs and are those needs that are given greater prominence and weight through social and political processes.

Next, we will turn our attention to measuring health.

Comprehension and Discussion Questions

- Why is it important to define health? Who influences the definition of health in your society?
- What is an example of a situation in which a different definition of health may lead to different policies?
- What are the advantages and disadvantages of considering social well-being and happiness as part of health?
- What is the difference between health conditions, health needs and health priorities?
- This chapter proposes different criteria to define health conditions (objective and subjective, present and future, external and internal, multidimensional). Can you think of examples for each criterion? Discuss how adopting them may impact our understanding of health conditions.

- Do you agree that health needs are social constructs? Provide an example of something that only recently became considered a health need in your society, or something that used to be considered a health need but isn't anymore.
- What criteria would you use to define health priorities for your country?

Papers from Which This Chapter Is Adapted

Donabedian, A. 1973. *Aspects of Medical Care Administration: Specifying Requirements for Health Care.* Cambridge, MA: Harvard University Press, pp. 58–88.

Frenk, J. & Gómez-Dantés, O. 2014. Designing a framework for the concept of health. *Journal of Public Health Policy*, 35, 401–406.

Chapter 4 Conceptual Basis for Measuring Health

Learning Objectives

- Investigate the importance of measuring health.
- Grasp the main approaches to measuring the health of populations.
- Understand the key methodological challenges associated with those approaches.
- Be able to describe how health measurement influences priority setting and explore the challenges associated with this use.

4.1 Introduction

We discussed in Chapter 3 various definitions of health and explored how they influence our understanding of health and disease, as well as our assessment of health conditions, needs and priorities. In this chapter, we turn to the question of measurement: Why measure health? How can we measure and compare various health states? Is population health just the aggregation of individual health? We describe various approaches to measuring the health of populations, explaining their potential limitations and methodological challenges.

Those challenges are not abstract. In the later part of this chapter, we explore how health measurements are used for priority setting, and the potential ethical and practical risks and challenges this creates.

4.2 Why Measure Health?

Attempts to count populations date to ancient times. Regular censuses were conducted in early civilizations, including the Babylonian empire, the Roman Empire and the Han Dynasty in China (Thorvaldsen, 2018). Such censuses helped governments assess wealth, plan resource allocation and determine taxes. But it is only much later that officials started taking an interest not just in the size of their populations but also in their health. In seventeenth-century England, the City of London started compiling weekly "bills of mortality," tracking the number and causes of deaths, as an early warning system to detect the plague (Feinleib, 2014). In 1662, John Grant, a London tradesman often considered the father of modern statistics, published an analysis of those bills of mortality, providing the first known life table. Health statistics were born.

Since then, interest in collecting and comparing health data has grown exponentially. Life expectancy was adopted early on as a powerful marker of population health (McDowell, 2006). Differences in life expectancy between countries can be as wide as 30 years (United Nations, 2020). Such a gap reveals important information regarding how healthy a population is.

But measures of mortality are insufficient to provide a complete picture of health, especially considering the rise of chronic diseases in the twentieth century (see Chapter 6 on health dynamics). Measures of morbidity also need to be collected to understand not just what individuals die of, but also what makes them unhealthy when alive.[1] Indicators focused on prevalence or incidence of disease and injury, such as the percentage of people living with HIV at any given moment (prevalence) or the number of new cases of malaria each year (incidence), can provide useful information. However, these conventional indicators are not easy to compare and provide little information regarding the effects of a disease on people's overall health. That is the role of generic health measures.

Generic health measures are, at their simplest, methods that attempt to quantitatively capture the "overall" health of an individual. By reducing health to a single measure, they can facilitate comparison across members of a population, across diseases and across time.

Why are we interested in capturing such health measures? Several uses emerge (Hausman, 2015). First, in clinical settings, generic health measures can be helpful to assess the overall impact of an intervention on a given individual. Say you want to understand the impact that a new cancer treatment may have on a patient's health. You know the treatment can effectively slow down the cancer's spread, but that it also has severe, debilitating side effects that will make the patient's daily life difficult. How can you weigh these different impacts? The regular use of a generic measure of health, such as the 36-item short-form (SF-36) health status survey, can help in this endeavor, for example, by tracking how the drug impacts the patient over time (Garratt et al., 1993).

At the population level, generic measures are even more useful to make comparisons. Let's go back to the cancer treatment example but now imagine you are a clinical trial researcher. You know your treatment is efficacious in men and women but may lead to stronger side effects for women. How can you measure such differences? Generic health measures, especially when they combine morbidity and mortality, can provide you with a systematic way to appraise the overall impact of different treatments or of a similar treatment across different populations.

Finally, in recent years, generic health measures have also emerged to guide public policy and health systems research. Its most famous example, the Global Burden of Disease study, originated at the World Health Organization and is now housed with the Institute for Health Metrics and Evaluation in Seattle, USA (Institute for Health Metrics and Evaluation, 2013). It attempts to assess the overall health of the global population using a single generic health measure, the disability-adjusted life year (DALY), to jointly track morbidity and mortality data and their distribution over causes, populations and times. Although the effort is not without criticisms, such standardized information can help identify health inequalities, prioritize where focus – including financial focus – is most needed and understand whether policies improve population health over time. Finally, generic measures can help us differentiate between the health conditions, health needs and health priorities we discussed in Chapter 3.

[1] The *mortality* rate refers to the number of deaths out of the total number of individuals in a specific population. Mortality is basically another term for death. The *morbidity* rate refers to the burden of illness or disease in a specific population. Both are commonly used in health statistics to characterize the health of a population.

4.3 How Can We Measure Health?

Now that we have established why we want to measure health, we must turn to how we can do so. Contrary to height, weight or blood pressure, overall health cannot be directly measured but must rely on an indirect, step-by-step approach. Just like feelings or intelligence, we don't expect to capture the essence of health: we merely hope to approximate it.

Health measures can commonly be grouped into two broad categories: health expectancies and health gaps. Health expectancies are based on real-life tables. This means that they are sensitive to change over time and do not easily allow for comparison across countries. Health gaps, on the other hand, can be more easily aggregated as they all refer to an ideal norm, but one that remains subjective. Box 4.1 provides more details on how these generic health measures are constructed.

Regardless of how those measures are used though, they both present several challenges in the way they approximate health.

A first difficulty resides in our ability to *define* health, its domains and boundaries. We established in Chapter 3 that health should not be restricted to physical health but should also include mental health. We further discussed the pros and cons of conflating health with well-being or happiness. Efforts to assign values to different health states will necessarily reflect these subjective choices. For example, we could choose a minimalist approach that would only measure body functions, such as mobility or pain, regardless of the individual's ability to use such functions in his or her daily life. Or we could favor a

Box 4.1 Health expectancies and health gaps

- **Health expectancies:** These incorporate non-fatal health outcomes into health expectancy calculations to estimate the expected number of years to be lived in an equivalent of "full health." The most used health expectancy indicator is the health-adjusted life expectancy (HALE) (Mathers, 2003). The HALE is calculated starting with real-life tables, and the probable duration of disability due to disease or injury is subtracted (Sullivan, 1971).
- **Health gaps:** These look at mortality gaps and add to them time lived in health states worse than ideal health. There are many health gap measures, but the most widely used is the DALY mentioned earlier. One DALY corresponds to one year of healthy life lost. DALYs grouped by cause of disease or injury will include the sum of years of life lost (YLLs) and the losses due to years lived with disability (YLDs). When working out these measures, current conditions are compared with an ideal target to assess loss due to premature mortality. For example, let's say an ideal target is 70 years of healthy life. Now, let's imagine someone who develops cancer at 50, then dies at 60 years old. This person has lost 10 years of life between 60 and 70 years old. In addition, she has lived 10 years, between 50 and 60, in a sub-optimal state due to cancer. As explained in the next section, researchers assign values to these different states, called disability weights. In this case, let's say they established that a year lived with this cancer corresponds to a 50% reduction of health. In other words, the cancer is so painful or disabling that two years lived with cancer would be equivalent to only one healthy year. The number of DALYs lost to this cancer would be the number of YLLs + the number of YLDs, so in this case 10 + 10 * 0.5 = 15 DALYs.

maximalist approach that would conflate health with quality of life, happiness or well-being (Bowling, 2005). Today, most efforts to define and measure health states adopt an intermediate approach that incorporates some elements of social functioning to the extent that they are "within the skin," that is, they are not substantially determined by interactions between the individual and his or her environment (Murray, 2002).

A second difficulty lies in our ability to *measure* those health states. For example, should we measure performance (what one actually does) or capacity (what one could potentially do)? Some authors have argued that performance is a function of capacity but also opportunity and preference and that therefore capacity should be privileged when measuring health. You may, for instance, have the capacity to swim 100 meters, but not the opportunity (no body of water nearby) or preference to do so; yet the capacity would tell us something important about your health. Others argue that the "lived experience" of individuals should be considered (Murray, 2002). For example, being in good enough health to swim 100 meters may be more important for a tour guide living on an island or a fisherman than someone in an urban landlocked environment. Survey design challenges can also arise. For instance, observed performance or capacity may be different from self-reported measures. When using self-reported measures, the duration chosen may lead to different answers; for example, if we are capturing health at the present moment or as experienced in the last four weeks.

The choices we make about boundaries, capacity and performance have practical implications on how we measure health and health interventions. Box 4.2 uses mobility, an essential part of health, to illustrate how choices made when defining and measuring mobility affect our understanding of which interventions to prioritize.

In summary, these are more than conceptual debates. Those choices have practical implications on how we measure health, how we measure health interventions and ultimately which interventions we may favor as a society.

A third difficulty lies in our ability to *compare* health states. Hausman argues that while efforts such as the Global Burden of Disease study[2] intend to measure health, they only really measure our *valuation* of health. In other words, when we compare someone with a common cold to someone with cancer, we are not saying that the person with the cold has more "health," but only that it is a preferable state (Hausman, 2015). How and who should decide on these preferences? If we design a scale, with 0 being full health and 1 being death, how can we position health states as different as being blind versus having back pain along this continuum? How can we compare chronic conditions over time with acute events? Are there conditions worse than death, such as extreme, unrelenting pain? Not only are those difficult choices to make, they are also very personal. What one person considers to be good health may differ from another person, depending on their age, personal background, cultural context or personal definition of health. In addition, no one can experience all health states, meaning researchers are forced to choose between asking specific patients about their own experience or asking the general public based on abstract situations (Helgesson et al., 2020).

Furthermore, researchers may struggle to consider the dynamic nature of health in these valuations. When it comes to disability, for example, research has shown that

---

[2] The Global Burden of Disease study is an initiative led by the Institute for Health Metrics and Evaluation since the 1990s, which estimates DALYs from hundreds of diseases, injuries and risk factors across the world.

Box 4.2 Boundaries, capacity and performance: the example of mobility

How we measure the impact of interventions on mobility will depend on how we have defined mobility in the first place:

- **Health boundaries:** Depending on whether we adopt a maximalist or minimalist definition of health, our definition of impact will differ. For example, if we adopt a "within the skin" definition of health, we will all agree that the health of a person with paraplegia who recovers the use of their legs after surgery has improved. But if this person is given a removable prothesis or relocates to a place more accessible for people with disabilities, we may not count those to be health improvement, even if the person's life has improved.
- **Capacity versus performance:** Similarly, how we measure health impact will depend on whether we decided to use capacity or performance as a proxy for health. For example, the surgeon may examine a person's legs and determine that they have the capacity to walk after surgery. But this person may not feel like walking, maybe because they fear falling. If we adopted a definition of health purely based on physical capacity, we may count this as a health improvement even if the person does not benefit from it.
- **Observed versus reported:** Finally, the way this information is captured may influence how impact is understood. Here, the most effective would be to observe people walking, but this might not always be feasible. So, a health researcher may instead ask people about their habits. If they ask this person whether they *can* walk, this person will answer yes. But if the health researchers asked them how often they walked in the last week or the last day, they may reply none. Clearly, the way the question is framed could lead to very different results.

individuals tend to adapt to their new situation and rebound back to reporting levels of well-being, particularly mental well-being, similar to those experienced prior to their disability (Grosse et al., 2009). The disability paradox also highlights a similar notion in describing how people living with disabilities may personally report a high quality of life, arguably in contrast to how others would perceive their state of health (Albrecht and Devlieger, 1999). Neglecting these realities would mean dismissing the lived experiences of people with disabilities, but incorporating them in health valuations could limit the importance we give to these conditions. At present, DALYs calculations are based on disability weights, which position different health outcomes along perfect health (0) to death (1). Various techniques are used to elicit preferences, including paired comparisons, person and time trade-off and standard gamble, with a vast literature discussing the strengths and flaws of each method.

Finally, we need to choose how we consider *time* when building health measures. A first choice relates to how we view health outcomes that will occur in the future versus those that occur in the present. Discounting, that is, placing a lower value on future outcomes compared to present ones, is common in economic evaluations of specific interventions. However, it presents specific challenges when applied at the population level. For example, disease eradication programs, such as for polio or smallpox, yield enormous benefits to future generations. Nevertheless, they may have little impact on present populations. Ultimately, choosing to apply or not a discounting rate to future generic health measures may paint very different pictures of the same disease burden.

Similarly, there has been extensive debate on whether DALYs should be weighted depending on the person's age when experiencing the disease or injury (Murray, 2002). These discussions implicitly assume that a year of life lost is not equal depending on whether you experience it at age 1, 25 or 97. In earlier iterations of DALYs, age weighting was applied to favor those between 9 and 54 years, on the justification that those individuals were primary caregivers. Age weighting has since been abandoned.

4.4 Using Generic Health Measures for Priority Setting

In Section 4.3, we discussed the many methodological challenges that arise when building generic health measures. These questions may appear as mere technicalities, but they are not trivial. In effect, choices made at each stage of this process can lead to very different valuations of health states. For example, Vigo and co-authors have argued that the Global Burden of Disease study may underestimate the burden of mental illness by more than a third (Vigo et al., 2016).

4.4.1 The Case for Priority Setting

This brings us back to our earlier point about why we care about generic health measures. At the population level, generic health measures can be a valuable resource for priority setting, that is, the strategic process through which we decide which health interventions or services to provide and in which order of importance. Formally or informally, this process happens across all settings, since resources allocated to health are de facto limited. But the criteria set to establish priorities are not always explicit and may vary over time. Health expectancies and gaps, capacity of the health system, funding availability, equity, urgency, the cost of inaction, etc. are all valid criteria to allocate resources, depending on societal values and concerns at any given moment. The COVID-19 pandemic is a good example of such criteria. While the burden of disease caused by the virus at the start of 2020 was relatively low, the estimated future impact and accompanying cost of inaction led health systems to prioritize responding to the crisis.

At its simplest, priority setting is about two criteria: magnitude of the problem – how large the burden is from the disease or injury – and potential for impact – how amenable the problem is to amelioration by an intervention. Generic health measures can provide useful information to estimate the magnitude of health problems and allocate resources accordingly.

4.4.2 Pitfalls and Challenges of Using Generic Health Measures for Priority Setting

Today, generic health measures are ubiquitous. Many countries explicitly use them to determine essential benefit packages or as part of the approval process for medicines and other technologies. Nevertheless, important ethical questions regarding their use remain. We will summarize four important debates.

1. **Scarcity and health care rationing:** A first question relates to whether such approaches should even be considered in the first place. Priority-setting methods assume that resources are scarce, and therefore, that distribution rules must be found. Human rights advocates, such as physician and anthropologist Paul Farmer, have argued that these discussions lead to a process of "socialization for scarcity" which, by

creating a narrative of resource scarcity, leads to sub-standard care for groups that have been socially marginalized (Farmer, 2004). This framing has been useful to push for broader resources for health and to unpack biases at play in resource allocation mechanisms, especially at the global level.

2. **Fairness and distributive justice:** A second debate relates to the extent to which using generic measures of health for resource allocation sufficiently incorporates considerations of fairness, equity and distributive justice. Generic measures of health such as those described in this section provide a utilitarian approach to health, with an implicit aim of "health maximization," meaning that choices should be made to maximize the total health of the population. However, adopting such a stance blurs who gets to experience such states. For example, generic health measures provide no guidance on what the philosopher Norman Daniels has called the "aggregation problem," that is, the idea that small, aggregated benefits across many individuals may ultimately yield many more health benefits than big benefits across only a few individuals, potentially yielding an unfair distribution of health care resources (Brock, 2010). Similarly, they also provide limited help to decide whether those worst off, for example, the sickest patients, should be given priority. Ultimately, equity and efficiency might not always be compatible, so policy-makers need to consider generic measures alongside other considerations of fairness and justice. (We discuss these concepts again in Chapters 5 and 7.)
3. **Population health as an aggregate of individual health:** A third issue relates to our conception of health as an individual attribute. Current methods to measure health are based on the implicit idea that health is first and foremost the attribute of an individual person. Therefore, the health of a population is an aggregate of individual measures of health. This idea underpins all the generic health measures described above. While essential, this approach alone is insufficient: it is not enough to simply aggregate the health status of the members of the population to fully characterize health in a population. We must also understand the way those members relate among themselves and how they relate to their environment, since the arrangements that structure such relationships determine the unequal distribution of health outcomes among the members of a population. In other words, in alignment with recent developments in complexity theory and system dynamics, one must consider that systems are more than the sum of their parts. Therefore, to get a precise and complete picture of the health of a population, one cannot simply focus on "dismantling it and examining its component parts"; efforts must also be made to understand how these parts connect and interact (McDowell et al., 2004). Adopting this comprehensive view of population health pushes us to explicitly consider how upstream systemic and structural factors affect individual health. For example, demographers have hotly debated why mortality improvements stalled or, in the case of the United States, degraded in the 2010s. One of the explanations for the United Kingdom appears to be the impact of austerity reforms on government spending (Hiam et al., 2018; Murphy et al., 2019). While it is likely such trends are due to a variety of factors, they shine a light on the relevance of broader economic policies to health.
4. **Population health and sustainability:** Finally, several analyses, such as the report of the Rockefeller Foundation–Lancet Commission on planetary health, argue that, while health measures like life expectancy (or DALYs) are helpful to measure the

health of those alive today, they fail to measure the impact of climate change on future generations or even our potential extinction, giving us a false sense of reassurance (Whitmee et al., 2015).

These four debates highlight the complexity researchers and policy-makers face when trying to measure health. Ultimately, though, it is not a matter of either/or. Our ability to combine those approaches – individual health measures, considerations of fairness and equity and broader measures of population health – is essential to gain a comprehensive understanding of the full complexity of this topic, which is a necessary condition to develop effective policies and practices.

4.5 Summary

Measuring health, much like defining it, is a complex endeavor, especially when trying to adopt a comprehensive approach capturing the "overall" health of an individual, as has been the case in recent decades. Developing generic health measures is useful to guide clinical and research decisions, and they are increasingly used at the population level for priority setting and resource allocation. However, researchers face numerous methodological trade-offs when developing those measures. They must adequately define the boundaries of health, then decide how to measure the multiple facets of health, how to compare various health states, and how to compare health states across individuals and across time. Considering these challenges, it is not surprising that the use of generic health measures, particularly for population-level decision-making, has been intensely debated. Recent developments in this field have focused on ethical considerations around fairness and equity, and on how to better incorporate broader determinants of health into current measures of population health. The latter topic is examined in detail in Chapter 5.

Comprehension and Discussion Questions

- Give at least three reasons why we measure health.
- What is the main difference between health expectancies and health gaps measures? What are the pros and cons of each approach?
- This chapter describes several methodological challenges linked to measuring health. Pick one of these challenges and explain how it applies to measuring a health topic of your choice.
- Do you think health measures should be used for priority setting? Why or why not?

Chapter 5

Determinants of Health

Learning Objectives

- Identify the different types of determinants of health and describe the scope and boundaries within which they exist.
- Specify the interrelationships between those factors and the levels at which they operate to drive health change.
- Explain the relationships between determinants, individual susceptibility and disease(s).
- Relate the concept of health determinant with health equity.

5.1 Introduction

In this chapter and Chapter 6, we move from defining health and identifying its domains, to understanding its dynamics – in other words, how health conditions change.

Health processes are always dynamic. Since the appearance of the first humans, people have interacted with the physical environment and other species. Human health has been affected by droughts and flooding, temperature fluctuations, animal diseases and the rise and extinction of predator species. The natural environment has also been transformed through the social organization of human populations. Against the background of their genetic make-up, the relationship of humans to others and to the natural environment has determined the appearance and disappearance of different diseases.

The concept of health transitions includes both the **transformation** of health conditions, which we will cover in Chapter 6, and the **determinants** of health status, which we cover in this chapter. To understand the factors that drive health change, we must first account for factors that determine health at any point in time. In this chapter, we propose a conceptual scheme that attempts to identify those factors, while specifying their interrelationships in a hierarchical framework of causality where multiple factors operate at different levels of determination. The final link in this chain is the individual, in whom disease processes express themselves. As we will argue, higher levels of determination impose structural limits to variation in lower levels. After specifying the scope of the overall framework, we explore the relationships between its various components, and the way they help explain the pathways between health and disease. We conclude this chapter with a discussion on equity in health and how it relates to determinants of health.

5.2 Framework Overview

There is a growing consensus that health and disease are determined in a multicausal way (Dubos, 1959; Black, 1980; Rothman, 1986; Putnam and Galea, 2008), and that they need to be approached from a comprehensive and interdisciplinary perspective. In order to do so, it is necessary to integrate the multiple determinant factors into a coherent analytical framework. Several attempts have been made to identify and elucidate such factors (Mosley and Chen, 1984; Cornia et al., 1987; Lynch et al., 2001; Marmot, 2006; Raphael, 2006; Kronenfeld, 2019; Dalsania et al., 2022). The framework we propose next tries to organize conceptually the complex multicausality of health conditions and systems. This framework is summarized in Figure 5.1, where the main relationships between health and its determinants are outlined. We will not attempt to examine thoroughly each of those relationships, nor will we review the available empirical evidence pertaining to them. Instead, we will concentrate on the basic conceptual aspects.

5.3 Scope of Analysis

We begin by deciding the scope and boundaries in which health and its determinants interact. The starting point in Figure 5.1 is the relationship between the population and its physical environment. From the standpoint of health determination, the most important population attributes are size, growth rate, age structure and geographic distribution. With respect to the environment, altitude, climate, natural resources and types of parasites and vectors exert important influences for specific disease processes. In addition, the long-term shifts in temperatures and weather patterns induced by the burning of fossil fuels since the eighteenth century generate important changes in the relationships between the population and its environment, both through radical changes in environmental risks and also through their impact on human societies, including forced migrations, change in food systems and exposure to extreme weather events.

Population and environment are linked through two major connectors. The first one is social organization, through which human beings develop the necessary structures and processes to transform nature (Commission on Social Determinants of Health, 2008). An example of such relationships is the role that urbanization plays in shaping the nature of the human habitat. The second connector is represented by the genome, which transforms the deepest constitution of human populations in response to changes in the environment. An example of this relationship is the sickle cell trait, a genetic modification which confers protection from severe malaria to those who bear it, and which is largely believed to be an example of natural genetic selection in areas with high malaria prevalence (Aidoo et al., 2002).

These four elements (population, environment, social organization and genome) set the broadest limits for the analysis of health determination. Indeed, all health phenomena occur in a population whose members have a certain genetic constitution and organize themselves socially to transform the environment. Specific relationships of determination take place within this basic frame.

5.4 Relationships between Components

We now aim to clarify the relationships between health outcomes and its determinants. Our conceptual formulation does not assume a diffuse multicausality, where everything

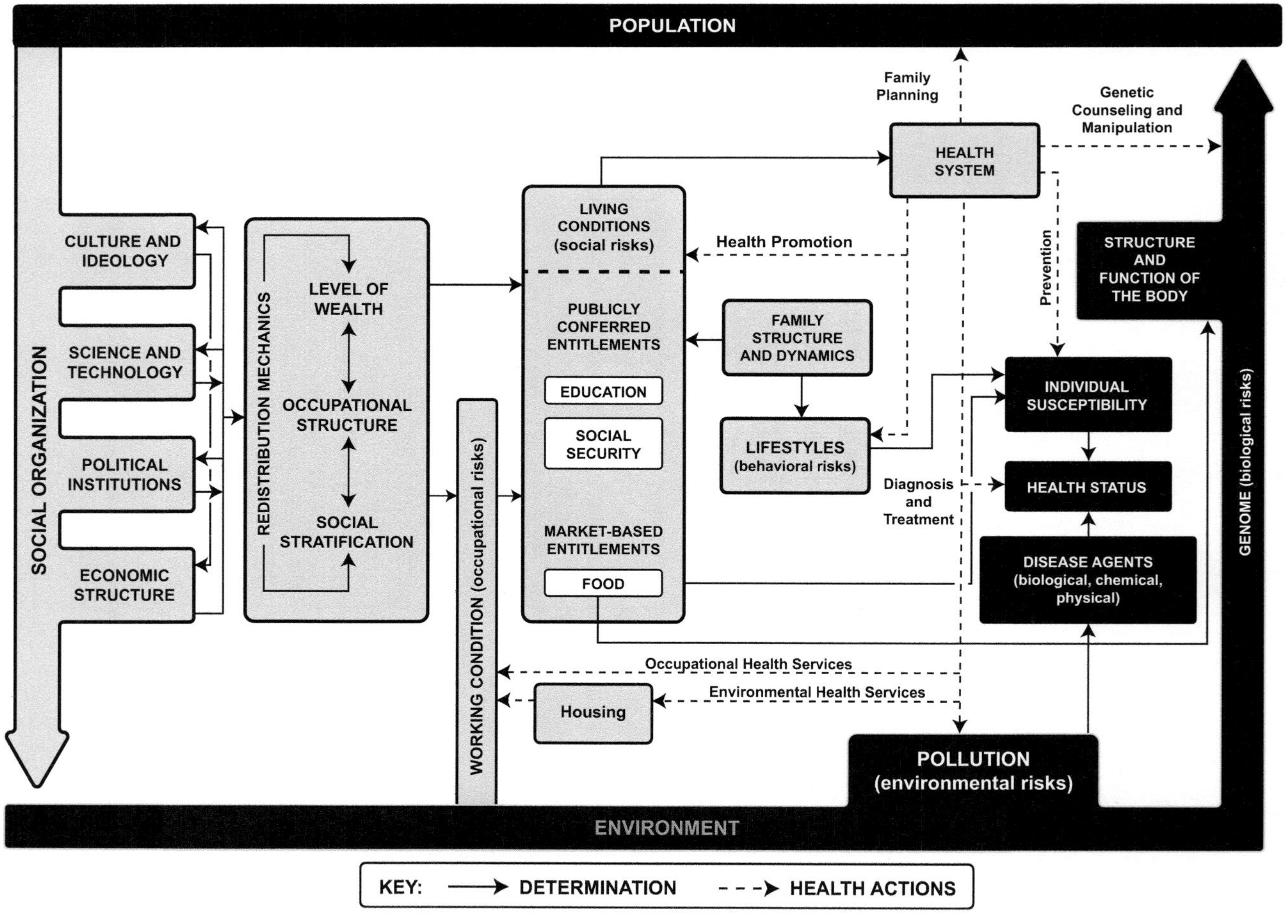

Figure 5.1 The determinants of health. From Frenk, J., Bobadilla, J. L., Stern, C., Frejka, T. & Lozano, R. (1991). Elements for a theory of the health transition. *Health Transition Review*, 1, 21–38.

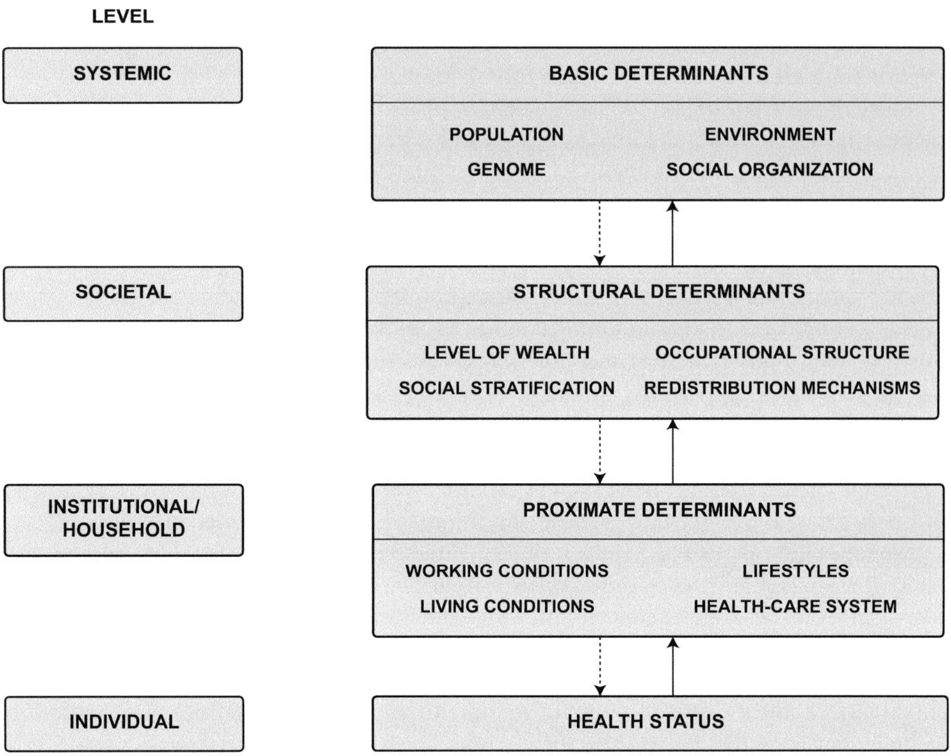

Figure 5.2 Types of determinants and levels of analysis in health. From Frenk, J., Bobadilla, J. L., Stern, C., Frejka, T. & Lozano, R. (1991). Elements for a theory of the health transition. *Health Transition Review*, 1, 21–38.

influences everything. Instead, it arranges determinants according to a hierarchy; this principle is schematized in the right-hand side of Figure 5.2, which summarizes the main relationships proposed in Figure 5.1, and includes arrows to define levels of determination along a feedback loop (the latter noted by the dotted arrows pointing up).

This conceptualization differs from other frameworks, such as McMahon's classic epidemiological "web of causation," which assumes no hierarchy between web nodes (MacMahon, 1970; Krieger, 1994). While this does not suggest per se a hierarchy of impact, it clearly posits that upper levels constrain lower levels, which has important implications for policy and practice.

5.5 Risk and Probabilities within the Model

At this point, it is necessary to highlight the central position given to the category of **risk** in our analysis. Risk is defined by Last as "a probability that an event will occur, e.g., that an individual will become ill or die within a stated period of time or age" (Last, 1983). For the purposes of this book, health determinants can be conceived of as risk factors, that is to say, processes, attributes or exposures that determine the probability of occurrence of disease or other health outcomes.

Furthermore, a dynamic conception cannot be restricted to visualizing an ideal state of health and a state of disease as the two extremes of a continuum (Terris, 1975);

instead, it must incorporate the various gradations within the continuum, that is, the risk levels. The complex interaction among basic, structural and proximate determinants (Figure 5.2) defines a whole spectrum of risk levels.

Since the concept of risk indicates a certain **probability** of suffering a loss of health, it necessarily refers to population groups (which offer the denominators for estimating probabilities). At a given moment, a high-risk situation may experience a change of state and bring about a health loss. It is in this step between risk and loss that the individual dimension of health is realized. Indeed, the population attribute of risk is translated, at the individual level, into a corresponding attribute that might be called "susceptibility" to disease agents. As Figure 5.1 shows, susceptibility is an individual attribute where working conditions, living conditions and lifestyles – determined by social processes – converge with body structure and function, as determined by biological processes. The case of COVID-19, presented in Chapter 14, clarifies this idea of susceptibility as an attribute defined by the convergence of social and biological determinants. Those most likely to develop symptoms and experience severe disease included both persons in vulnerable social circumstances, such as essential workers who could not work remotely, and persons with pre-existing medical conditions who were immunocompromised.

Susceptibility is also a product of the interaction between the internal and the external milieus, the balance of which determines health, according to Dubos and other advocates of the ecological conception. Thus, the transformation of the environment by human beings generates pollution, understood in a broad sense as the presence of biological, chemical and physical agents that may act upon susceptible individuals and potentially produce disease. It should be noted that this broad definition of pollution includes not only the active introduction into the environment of disease agents as a result of human activity but also the failure to remove agents that occur naturally.

This conception of risk is in no way static. The concept of **life course**, first proposed by Kuh and Ben-Shlomo in 1997 and widely adopted since, is relevant to this framework. The life course posits that relationships between the individual and his or her environment should be envisioned longitudinally, as experiences earlier during gestation, birth or childhood will influence individual health later in life (Kuh and Ben-Shlomo, 2004; Kelly et al., 2009). An individual's experiences in childhood, for example, can become "embodied" and impact his or her risk and susceptibility later in life. For example, numerous studies have shown how birth weight can impact health later in life, regardless of the individual's subsequent experience (Hack et al., 1995; Gamborg et al., 2009).

5.6 Pathways to Health and Disease

In order to analyze these relationships in greater detail, it is convenient to start from the left side of Figure 5.1, which focuses on the social determinants. As can be seen, there are four major dimensions of social organization: economic structure; political institutions; science and technology; and culture and ideology. Together, these dimensions determine the total level of wealth of a society and the rules for stratifying different groups. Two major factors mediate the differential access of those groups to the total wealth pool: on the one hand, the occupational structure; on the other, the redistribution mechanisms utilized by the State, notably taxes and subsidies.

It is beyond the scope of this book to elaborate on the complex relationship among these various categories, which is the subject of many of the most lasting and profound debates in the social sciences. For our purposes, suffice it to say that these elements constitute the structural determinants of the health and disease process. Together, they constrain the variation of a set of proximate determinants, namely, working conditions, living conditions, lifestyles and the health care system (see Figure 5.2).

Lifestyle is a behavioral manifestation of beliefs, information and the constraints within which people live. The access to information that shapes beliefs and lifestyles has changed radically with the advent of the internet and social media. In the past, the challenge was access. Now, it's a problem of curation, of making sense of the information and, increasingly, of identifying and selecting trustworthy information.

The separation between working and living conditions is, of course, arbitrary. The purpose is to highlight the critical importance of work both as a direct determinant of the worker's health status and as an indirect contributor to the health of the rest of the family. In recognition of its direct effect, working conditions are portrayed in Figure 5.1 as part of the worker's immediate environment. Such an effect is due to the occupational risks that derive from working conditions.

As shown in Figure 5.1, living conditions occupy a central position among the proximate determinants of health. In turn, living conditions depend mainly on what the philosopher Amartya Sen calls the "exchange entitlement" of an individual or family, that is, the alternative bundles of goods and services that the individual can acquire in exchange for what he or she owns (Sen, 1981). For our present purpose, it is very important to distinguish two types of entitlements, according to whether they are publicly conferred or market based. This distinction depends on the rules governing access to goods and services. Simply stated, market-based entitlements can be obtained by exchanging money, labor or goods for other goods and services, in a manner governed by the logic of the market. In contrast, publicly conferred entitlements are goods and services that, through the intervention of some collective actor – generally the State – are removed from market distribution and made available either as a supplement to market exchange or as a social right; they are considered as a requisite for equality of opportunity, which provides the ethical foundation for market competition (Briggs, 1961). For example, in many countries, governments provide primary and secondary education to all residents free of charge as a publicly conferred entitlement and funded through taxation; in some countries, tertiary (university-level) education, however, is treated as a market-based entitlement that must be purchased.

It is not enough for the State to declare certain goods or services to be a social right; it is necessary to analyze the extent to which such a declaration is put into practice (Ruger, 2006; Panjwani and Caraher, 2014). In many countries, for example, South Africa, health (including access to health care) is a human right guaranteed by the national constitution (Kinney and Clark, 2004). However, the extent to which it is realized varies widely between urban and rural areas, and realizing this right is understood to be progressive as the State cannot immediately ensure access for every resident to all necessary goods and services (Gaede and Versteeg, 2011). The distinction between market-based and publicly conferred entitlements varies across time and among societies. Furthermore, access to the same goods (e.g., certain food) may be governed by the market for some social groups but by the State for others (e.g., those earning less than a specified minimum). Despite these complexities, it is possible, in almost all circumstances, to make this distinction.

Within the sphere of market-based entitlements, food and housing are of special interest due to their effects on health (McKeown, 1976, Kushel et al., 2006). Among other elements, food intake involves nutrition, which conditions biological development and thus affects the structure and function of the body, including its resistance to infection and also its susceptibility to chronic diseases. For example, recent studies on the link between ultra-processed food and obesity reveal the important role that nutrition plays in shaping health status (Askari et al., 2020; Gomes Gonçalves et al., 2023). In turn, housing is represented in Figure 5.1 as a bridge between living conditions and the environment, since it constitutes the immediate habitat of human beings. Moreover, while a house in good condition may be a protection against environmental risks, poor housing conditions (e.g., lead in water pipes or asbestos in building materials) add to deleterious environmental factors because they too are sources of pollution (Krieger and Higgins, 2002). Among the principal elements that link housing with the environment are water supply and sanitation, which are important determinants of health (Shuval et al., 1981; Montgomery and Elimelech, 2007; Fink et al., 2011; World Health Organization, 2022a). The COVID-19 pandemic has also highlighted the importance of indoor air pollution and ventilation, including in the transmission of pathogens (Agarwal et al., 2021).

In terms of health effects, education and social security stand out among the most important publicly conferred entitlements. In particular, women's education has been shown to be a critical factor in child health, although the precise mechanism through which this effect is exerted remains a matter of debate (Desai and Alva, 1998; Victora et al., 2011; Bado and Sathiya Susuman, 2016; Perkiö, 2021). With respect to formal social security systems, it is convenient, for the purposes of this book, to distinguish them from health care services, even though in many countries a single institution may be responsible for both. Strictly speaking, social security services refer to benefits that assure minimum levels of economic and social well-being. They include social insurance services, considered as economic and social fringe benefits for workers who contribute to premiums, as well as social assistance services for vulnerable persons who are not required to pay health insurance premiums, or even health services. Examples of such assistance include food vouchers, temporary income in case of unemployment and cash transfers for the care of children.

It is necessary to point out that, apart from being a means for redistributing access to certain goods and services, publicly conferred entitlements also have economic, political and ideological value. In an economic sense, they represent a means for the survival of large sectors of the population. They also have a political value in a double sense: on the one hand, they are the object of demands by social groups; on the other, they are means to exercise political control. In this last sense, the ideological value of entitlements must also be understood as a way of legitimizing a social system. These multiple values explain, at least in part, the unequal character of publicly conferred entitlements in many countries, which often contradicts the declared universality of access to them. Hence, these entitlements – notably social insurance – have been mainly directed toward groups involved in the formal sector of the economy, where the aforementioned values can be more effectively realized. As we will see when we discuss health reforms, a big part of the political agenda in recent years has been to expand those entitlements beyond salaried workers.

As indicated earlier, the summation of market-based and publicly conferred entitlements defines living conditions. Through the mediation of family structure and dynamics, living conditions affect the next proximate determinant of health status, namely, lifestyles. Lifestyles are also directly affected by culture and ideology, as well as laws, regulations, taxes, subsidies and the pressures of commercial enterprises (though these relationships are not portrayed in Figure 5.1 for reasons of simplification). As Coreil et al. have argued, the notion of lifestyle has gained wide currency in the health field without an adequate conceptual analysis. The most common usage reduces its meaning to specific individual behaviors that are interpreted as risk factors (Coreil et al., 1985). This usage does not take proper account of the sociocultural context of behavior, which was central to the original sociological meaning of lifestyle. Coriel et al. propose that this concept be applied to behaviors that are shared by a social group in a specific context. In this sense, it represents a conceptual bridge between cultural and behavioral patterns.

In accordance with this broader perspective, Figure 5.1 makes a fundamental distinction between living conditions and lifestyles. The former refers to the objective material situation in which the different social groups exist; the latter represents the way in which those social groups translate their objective situation into patterns of behaviors. Therefore, living conditions generate what could be called "social risks," while lifestyles produce "behavioral risks." Considered as a whole, both define the quality of life. Undoubtedly, an exhaustive conceptual development will require an operationalization of the categories of living conditions and lifestyles. However, for the time being, it suffices to establish their position in the determination of health status.

In a feedback loop of determination, the health system may, in its turn, influence: (1) the basic and structural determinants (by means of family planning, environmental health services and genetic counseling); (2) the proximate determinants (by means of occupational health services and health promotion); (3) individual susceptibility (through primary preventive actions, such as vaccinations); and (4) health status once it has been determined (through diagnostic and therapeutic services). It is important to point out that this influence can be both positive and negative. Medical errors, bias, stigma or the provision of sub-quality care can all negatively impact the health status of patients.

The complete set of processes included in our theoretical framework can be summarized as portrayed in Figure 5.2. A fundamental element of the framework is that, as shown on the left side of this figure, five analytical levels can be distinguished: systemic, societal, institutional, household and individual. (Figure 5.2 visually shows four levels, since we combine institutional and household.) The systemic and societal levels correspond to the basic and structural determinants, respectively. In turn, the proximate determinants can be analyzed at two levels: the social institutions that give them an organizational expression and the family processes that articulate their expression in the household (DaVanzo, 1990). Finally, health status is defined, as mentioned earlier, at the individual level. From top to bottom, each analytical level "explains" (or sets the limits of variability of) the factors operating at the level below; from bottom to top, "explanations" of elements at each level (or the limits of actual existing alternatives) must be sought through the characteristics and operation of factors from levels above.

This figure should be seen simply as a schematic device to portray the notion of hierarchical multicausality that underlies our theoretical framework. In no way does the figure suggest that the higher analytical levels are intrinsically more important or complex than the lower ones. On the contrary, many of the conceptual breakthroughs in explaining and improving health status will come from a better understanding of the subtle interactions operating at the institutional, household and individual levels. Furthermore, our formulation does not imply a unidirectional flow of determination. While the solid arrows in Figure 5.2 do postulate a dominant direction of determination, the dotted arrows illustrate the existence of important feedback loops. The COVID-19 pandemic was a real-life illustration of the subtle ways through which these determinants influenced one another and, ultimately, individual susceptibility to the virus. A more detailed analysis of these interactions with respect to the pandemic is presented in Chapter 14.

5.7 Determinants of Health and Equity

Debates related to determinants of health are intimately linked to discussions of equity and justice. This is quite natural: the same way that health outcomes are unequally distributed across the population, so are all those determinants. Understanding which factors drive health change and how such factors are distributed across the population can help us address them and ultimately impact health. As we will see later in Chapter 7, health systems aim to improve the absolute level of health of a given population, but also its distribution across groups and individuals. In order to do so, policy-makers need to understand the factors accounting for unequal distribution patterns.

The concepts of equality and equity play pivotal roles in this understanding, including in the realms of research, practice, assessment and organization within the health care system. Equality refers to ensuring everyone has the same resources or opportunities, while equity is concerned with fairness and justice, aiming for proportional distribution based on individual needs. These distinctions are crucial to consider in public health, as disparities can arise from various social, economic and cultural determinants. Analytical tools such as the Gini coefficient and the Lorenz curve are useful to evaluate inequality by summarizing the distribution of a variable and its deviation from perfect equality. Methods designed to estimate equity in a population strive to guide the fair allocation of resources on two dimensions: horizontal equity, meaning equal treatment of those with equal needs, and vertical equity, which proposes higher levels of care for people with greater needs. The latter implies that it is fair to provide unequal treatment to people with unequal needs (Raine et al., 2016).

Not all differences between individuals matter equally when considering pathways to disease and determinants of health, neither do they lead to similar responses. Both reflect societal choices and values.

Often, researchers and public health practitioners will consider individual elements that extend across all levels of analysis, building upon the interconnectivity among all determinants of health. For example, race as a mediating factor in public health presents a pathway that includes determinants and outcomes from the systems to the individual level. Racism contributes to health disparities and is recognized as a major driver in the disproportionate levels of morbidity and mortality among Black individuals, for example, or Indigenous people (Gee and Ford, 2011). Structural racism is generally regarded as a feature of society that reflects the system of policies, practices and cultural norms perpetuating racial inequity (Aspen Institute, 2017). This concept illustrates how historical developments enable racism and discrimination to persist in contemporary society, causing adverse health outcomes in various populations. Essentially, the legacy of

Box 5.1 Determinants of maternal mortality in the United States

The United States has the highest rate of maternal mortality among high-income countries (HICs), with 22 maternal deaths for every 100,000 live births in 2022. This rate is two to three times higher than most other HICs. Stark differences exist between races, with maternal mortality being significantly higher for Black women (49.5 per 100,000 live births) compared to White (19.0), Hispanic (16.9) and Asian (13.2) women (Hoyert, 2022).

At the individual level, underlying health conditions, such as hypertension or diabetes, can help explain those deaths. But focusing on biomedical markers or lifestyle risk factors only would miss the forest for the trees. Racial disparities persist even when those risk factors are not present.

At the proximate level, access to high-quality reproductive and maternal health services, financial protection and health insurance, access to paid parental leave, food stability and housing, among other factors, also play an important role.

Even after controlling for underlying social and economic factors, such as education and income, inequalities still persist. This is why it is critical to take into account structural factors, such as historical exposure to racial trauma, discrimination or implicit bias in the health care system.

slavery, colonialism and racially motivated discrimination has left lasting impacts on many members of society today.

Bailey et al. analyze the way in which factors relating to race in the United States moderate the role of social determinants on health outcomes through three domains: redlining and racialized residential segregation; mass incarceration and police violence; and unequal medical care (Bailey et al., 2021). Historically grounded discrimination has forced the existence of these domains, and the interrelated elements of each push compounded consequences through each level of analysis.

Just as race is a mediating factor in the example above, understanding each respective determinant in public health is essential for developing targeted and equitable interventions. Health outcomes are influenced by a complex interplay of factors, and the impact of these factors can vary among different population groups. By considering the complexities and interrelationships between determinants, levels of analysis and health outcomes, public health practitioners and researchers can develop more effective strategies to address health disparities and promote health equity.

The example in Box 5.1 concerning the determinants of maternal mortality in the United States shows the complex and interconnected pathways between determinants, risks and individual susceptibility. Understanding those pathways is key to designing solutions and addressing this unacceptable failure (Crear-Perry et al., 2021; Njoku et al., 2023).

5.8 Summary

This chapter has provided a conceptual framework to organize the complex relationships between multiple determinants that underlie changes in the health conditions of a population. Specific relationships of determination take place within a basic frame comprised of the population, its genetic constitution, the physical environment within which it resides and its forms of social organization. The multiple determinants at work within this frame operate at five hierarchically organized levels – systemic, societal, institutional, household and individual – with each analytical level limiting the variability of the factors operating at the level below. The complex interaction among determinants defines a spectrum of risk levels for the population that is translated into susceptibility to disease agents at the individual level, including throughout a person's life course.

The framework developed here allows us to appreciate the complex determination of health processes and identify areas for future research. In particular, each of the six revolutions mentioned in the final chapter of this book has the potential of modifying the determinants of health in the future.

This framework provides the basis to understand the dynamic way in which health conditions change over time, which is the subject of Chapter 6.

Comprehension and Discussion Questions

1. What is the difference between a health determinant and a health condition?
2. In Figure 5.2, we propose four levels of determinants. Choose a health condition and identify a determinant for it at each level. Explain the causal pathways between your determinant and the health condition.
3. In this chapter, we propose a conceptual framework based on "hierarchical multicausality," which we contrast against a "diffuse" causality model. What is the key difference between these two ideas, and why does it matter?
4. Using the same example from Question 2, highlight how the determinants you have described relate to one another using the concept of "hierarchical multicausality."
5. How do health determinants relate to individual risk and susceptibility?
6. Do you agree with the statement that "it is fair to provide unequal treatment to people with unequal needs"? Why or why not?

Papers from Which This Chapter Is Adapted

Frenk, J., Bobadilla, J. L., Stern, C., Frejka, T. & Lozano, R. 1991. Elements for a theory of the health transition. *Health Transition Review*, 1, 21–38.

Chapter 6

Health Dynamics: How Health Conditions and Needs Change

Learning Objectives

- Describe the megatrends in mortality, morbidity and economic development in the twentieth century.
- Relate those to the concept of the health transition, and explain its drivers and mechanisms.
- Distinguish between the concepts of health transition, demographic transition and epidemiological transition.
- Discuss the limitations and shortcomings of the concept of epidemiological transition, both across populations and contexts and in relationship with climate change.
- Apply the above concepts to upcoming challenges and trends.

6.1 Introduction

So far, we have examined the definition of health conditions and needs, as well as their dimensions and determinants. Now we need to understand them in a dynamic way, to analyze how they change.

This chapter presents the basic elements for developing a theory of the health transition. Such elements include the definition of concepts, the analysis of the mechanisms through which health change occurs in populations, the characterization of the attributes that allow us to identify different transition models and the enumeration of the possible consequences of the transition. This theory builds in part upon the vast transformations brought about by the demographic and epidemiological transitions observed during the twentieth century in most parts of the world. We attempt to explain the complexities – and in some case contradictions – of this vast transformation, and to explore how health outcomes may continue to change in the twenty-first century as underlying mechanisms evolve. The purpose is to derive propositions that can be generalized, providing a comprehensive theoretical basis for comparative studies of health dynamics, while acknowledging the specificity of each national reality at each historical moment. At the outset, it should be made clear that the health transition is a long-term process of change, not a specific period of time.

This chapter is divided into four sections. First, we describe the megatrends in mortality, morbidity and economic development during the twentieth century, which have led researchers to develop models of demographic and epidemiological transitions to explain these changes. Second, we use these transitions as a starting point to derive and systematize the main components of an epidemiological transition theory, while also pointing out its potential shortcomings and limitations. In the third section, we explore the attributes of such changes, in order to understand how these same underlying concepts can be applied to analyze different patterns of disease, disability and death across countries and among socioeconomic groups, as well as to understand emerging trends in the twenty-first century, such as stalling or declining life expectancy in some high-income countries, or the emergence of new infectious disease epidemics. Finally, we explore what the consequences of this epidemiological transition are on a broader health transition.

The last century has been one of unprecedented change. The only certainty today is an increasing complexity. Conceptual models can help make sense of this but are insufficient to give a full account of the complexity of several transition patterns observed within and among different countries. Therefore, we do not intend here to offer a finished theory, but rather some elements that will make progress in research and understanding possible.

6.2 The Three Revolutions of the Twentieth Century

Before describing a conceptual model of health transition, it is important to first describe three revolutions of the twentieth century, which underpin our conceptual understanding of the health transition.

The first revolution was the **demographic transition**, which is characterized by a shift from high birth rates and high death rates to low birth rates and low death rates. This process has been almost universally experienced, although under diverse patterns across different parts of the world (Chesnais, 1992).

The demographic transition was accompanied by the largest public health transition perhaps ever experienced: a dramatic change in life expectancy. For as far back as scientists can estimate, life expectancy remained relatively flat, due to high average levels of mortality, though there were periods of major increases in death rates leading to cataclysmic drops in life expectancy during outbreaks of the plague in Europe, for example, or when smallpox essentially destroyed the Aztec and Inca empires. In contrast, life expectancy at birth, as shown in Figure 6.1, more than doubled during the twentieth century, with an acceleration of this trend after World War II, until generalized reversals occurred in the aftermath of the COVID-19 pandemic (United Nations, 2022).

These dramatic changes had widespread and dramatic implications for public health, bringing both a quantitative jump as well as a qualitative shift in the nature of the dominant patterns of disease, disability and death in human populations. The **epidemiological transition**, the second one that spanned the twentieth century, involved, in turn, three major changes or megatrends:

- To begin with, there was a major shift in the **dominant causes of death**. Mostly, the direction goes from infectious to non-infectious diseases. The cause structure of mortality switched during the transition of the twentieth century. Infectious diseases lost their previous dominance, but still maintained a major position in the epidemiological profile. At the same time, the absolute and relative importance of non-communicable diseases increased. Apart from social inequality in the quantitative levels of mortality, there is now a qualitative inequality in the distribution of causes of death by geographical region and social class.

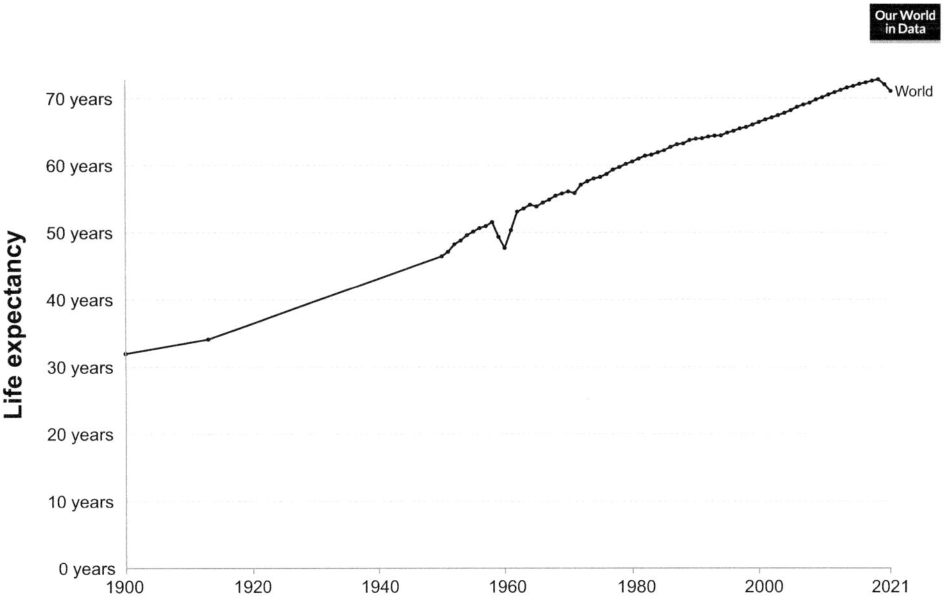

Figure 6.1 The doubling of life expectancy during the twentieth century. Adapted from Riley (2005), Zijdeman and Ribeira da Silva (2015), Human Mortality Database (2023) and United Nations (2024) – with minor processing by Our World in Data. The graph plots period life expectancy, which is a metric that summarizes death rates across all age groups in one particular year. For a given year, it represents the average lifespan for a hypothetical group of people, if they experienced the same age-specific death rates throughout their whole lives as the age-specific death rates seen in that particular year.

- The **age structure of mortality** also switched, from deaths concentrated in young people to more and more happening in the elderly, getting closer to the biological limits of life. That dramatic drop in mortality did not happen uniformly but was highly concentrated in the reduction of infant and child mortality, mostly from infectious diseases.
- The two previous changes lead to a fundamental shift in the **experience of disease**. For most of human history, the experience of disease was related to acute episodes from which you either die or recover only to later develop other episodes. You get sick from acute diarrhea; if you don't die from that, you recover and get malaria; and if you don't die from that, you go on to get something else. When you have acute episodes of disease, mortality dominates the health picture, with the central problem being the death of children. When the dominant disease pattern shifts to chronic conditions, such as cancer, diabetes or even HIV/AIDS, which thanks to access to antiretroviral therapy can persist for many decades, morbidity becomes more important in the epidemiological picture, as people spend long periods of time in less-than-perfect health. This has been a key facet of the ongoing transition in the twentieth century.

Finally, since the end of the nineteenth century, the world has experienced a deep economic and social transformation, linked to a dramatic increase in economic growth and energy consumption, both a cause and a consequence of the demographic and epidemiological transitions described above. Figure 6.2 shows in one glance the dramatic increase in gross domestic product (GDP) per capita experienced in the last two

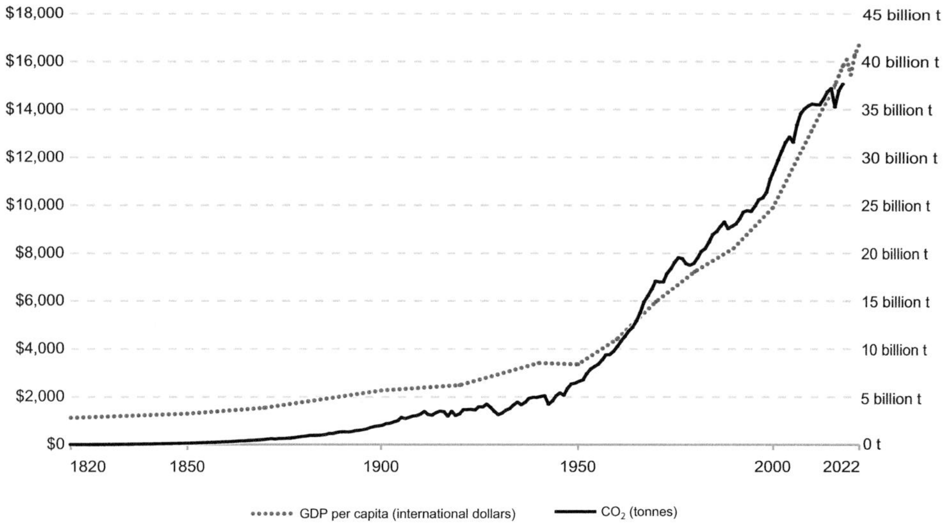

Figure 6.2 Increase in GDP per capita and carbon dioxide (CO_2) emissions worldwide, measured in US dollars and tonnes, respectively. Adapted from Bolt and van Zanden – Maddison Project Database 2023 – with minor processing by Our World in Data; Global Carbon Budget 2025 – with major processing by Our World in Data (https://archive.ourworldindata.org/20260119-070102/grapher/co2-intensity.html). CO_2 emissions are from fossil fuels and industry. Land-use change is not included. GDP per capita is a country's gross domestic product divided by its population. These data are adjusted for inflation and differences in living costs between countries.

centuries. It is beyond the scope of this book to analyze the underlying reasons for this transformation, including the Industrial Revolution, which started in Western Europe in the eighteenth century, and the rapid expansion of global trade during the last 40 years. Suffice it to say that this change in economic patterns was intrinsically linked to a change in energy consumption, particularly from fossil fuels, a powerful driver of economic growth. This has led to a significant human impact on Earth's geology and ecosystems, sometimes dubbed the age of the "Anthropocene" to denote the impact of human activities on Earth (Crutzen, 2002). The exploitation of Earth's natural resources has resulted in a significant disruption of ecosystems, which threatens to reverse the gains in life expectancy achieved during the twentieth century. As such, the epidemiological transition needs to be conceptualized and understood within the broader context of an evolving climate crisis.

6.3 Conceptual and Theoretical Base of the Health Transition

The three epidemiological megatrends described earlier have unfolded differently across contexts and countries. Nevertheless, their underlying characteristics can be useful to define a conceptual and theoretical base that allows us to arrange and give coherence to the growing body of empirical evidence in order to understand the dynamics of health change.

This section outlines the general elements needed to delve into the theory of the health transition:

1. **Concepts:** What is the definition of the object of analysis that the theory intends to account for?
2. **Mechanisms:** Which factors explain changes in the object?

3. **Attributes:** How is the object characterized?
4. **Consequences:** What effects does it have on other processes?

The rest of this section attempts to give a preliminary answer to each of the above questions as they relate to the health transition.

6.3.1 Concepts

After the classical writings of authors like Virchow, Malthus, Marx and Engels, an early attempt to analyze the health implications of demographic and economic transitions was published by Frederiksen more than 50 years ago (Frederiksen, 1969). In 1971, Omran coined the term "epidemiologic[al] transition" and thus made way for a major breakthrough in our understanding of the dynamics of causes of death in populations (Omran, 1971). Almost simultaneously, and apparently in an independent way, Lerner presented a paper postulating a "health transition," a broader concept than the one used by Omran, since it included elements of the social conceptions and behaviors regarding health determinants (Lerner, 1973).

While not many conceptualization and research activities were carried out during the decade that followed those pioneering works, there has been a renewed interest in the concept of the epidemiological transition after the 1990s, with many groups of researchers, national institutions and international agencies becoming interested in this concept as a way to attract political attention to the rise of non-communicable diseases in low-income and middle-income countries (Herrick, 2022).

Largely owing to this renewed interest, the concept of epidemiological transition has been given various meanings that need to be clarified. In particular, it is common to refer to the transition as a period more than as a process of change. In this first viewpoint, the epidemiological transition is regarded as a time interval, beginning when infectious diseases were predominant, and ending when non-communicable diseases finally dominated the causes of death.

Instead of this rather static perspective, we propose to conceive the transition as a dynamic process, in which the health and disease patterns of a society evolve in diverse ways as a response to broader demographic, socioeconomic, technological, political, cultural and biological changes. A transition is not just any change; it is change that follows an identifiable pattern and that occurs over a relatively long period of time. However, if we accept that health conditions are continuously being transformed – as different diseases disappear, appear or re-emerge – it can be stated that the transition is an ongoing process of change, rather than a relatively simple and unidirectional period of time. In addition, it also means that this transition can be truncated or even reversed.

Finally, one more cause of confusion often comes from including, in the definition of epidemiological transition, processes that constitute mechanisms through which the transition occurs. This confusion may be observed particularly with regards to fertility changes. Since the original work by Omran in 1971, there has been a tendency to include fertility decline as a defining element of the different epidemiological transition models (Omran, 1982). This tendency is even more explicit in a revision done later by Omran himself (Omran, 1983). As we try to demonstrate later, fertility decline is one of the main mechanisms through which prevailing morbidity and mortality patterns change but is not in itself part of the definition of the epidemiological transition.

6.3.2 Mechanisms

Health status is expressed at the individual level. Its aggregation defines the epidemiological profile of a population. And the long-term change in such a profile constitutes the epidemiological transition. Having specified in Chapter 5 the determinants of individual health status, a theory of the transition must also account for the mechanisms that drive change at the aggregate level.

Three major mechanisms are involved in the epidemiological transition (Mosley et al., 1990). Each of them also refers to long-term transformations. They are fertility decline, which alters the age structure of a population; changes in risk factors, which affect the incidence of diseases; and improvements in health care technology and organization, which modify case fatality rates (Figure 6.3).[1]

1. **Fertility decline:**[2] This process, part of the demographic transition, involves a shift from a situation where fertility is dominated by natural and biological factors to another in which fertility is controlled by the decisions of potential parents, themselves influenced by socioeconomic and cultural factors, such as women's participation in the workforce or societal perceptions around family size. As a result of fertility declines, societies fundamentally change their age structures. From a distribution biased toward young ages, they move to one in which adults predominate. Earlier in the demographic transition, the absolute number of adults increases due to population growth caused by a decrease in mortality combined with high fertility. Subsequently, when the latter declines, the adult population continues growing due to the aging of persons born under the past conditions of high fertility. At the same time, the relative preponderance of adults becomes evident, since the decline of fertility causes the number of new persons in the youngest ages to be smaller than would be the case with higher fertility.

   In epidemiological terms, the result of this process is an increase in the absolute number and the proportion of persons exposed to non-communicable diseases, such as cardiovascular problems and cancer. Thus, even with constant age-specific incidence rates, the absolute volume of patients and deaths resulting from this type of disease increases substantially. Moreover, the total number of deaths also rises due to the new age structure.
2. **Changes in risk factors:** Unlike the previous one, this mechanism acts primarily on the probabilities of becoming ill, that is, on the incidence of diseases. According to our analytical framework (see Chapter 5), the underlying force in the modification of such probabilities is the change in the various types of risks: biological, environmental, occupational, social and behavioral. In the twentieth century, many of those changes have been associated with the process of economic growth and the social and cultural changes associated with it. A detailed analysis of its social, economic and cultural dimensions is beyond the scope of this book. Nevertheless, it is

[1] The case fatality rate is the number of people who die due to a disease out of the total number of people diagnosed with the disease. Compared to the mortality rate, it does not take into account the time period between the disease onset and death. The case fatality rate provides a sense of how lethal the disease is.

[2] We should specify here that the term "fertility decline," commonly used in demography, refers to a decrease in birth rates, not a decrease in fertility per se.

worth mentioning the manifestations that most significantly influence health risks. Overall, they include the shift from a society dominated by agricultural production to one in which industrial production predominates, which also implies a notable increase in productivity. Closely related is the change in population distribution, from rural to predominantly urban settlements. These socioeconomic changes have occurred in parallel with two cultural transformations: the expansion of education, which provides access to a minimum level of schooling common to most members of society; and the increased participation of women in the labor force, which is related to profound modifications in the dynamics of families and communities.
An important condition accompanying these changes is the average improvement in nutrition, housing, water supply and sanitation, which significantly decreases health risks (McKeown, 1976; Evans et al., 1981).

From the point of view of the epidemiological transition, most economic, social and cultural changes usually associated with this economic transition have a double face: some help to reduce the incidence of infectious diseases and health risks related to reproduction; others generate an increase of non-communicable diseases and injury. For example, the introduction of basic urban infrastructure and the adoption of hygienic measures considerably reduce the incidence of infections. Also, the acceptance of effective contraceptive methods, which is associated with the increased participation of women in the labor force, not only decreases fertility levels but also alters reproduction patterns, for example, by extending time intervals between births. There is evidence that these modified patterns improve maternal and neonatal survival by reducing exposure to high-risk pregnancies (Fortney, 1987; Schlaepfer et al., 1990).

But not all aspects are positive. The working and living conditions of many urban dwellers produce a higher incidence of injuries. Similarly, the adoption of certain patterns of consumption and behavior increases the overall risk of becoming ill and dying. There is now extensive evidence on the impact of various risk factors, including the consumption of alcohol, cigarettes and unhealthy food, as well as the lack of physical activity, on the probability of developing non-communicable diseases. Environmental risk factors, including air pollution and exposure to toxic chemicals, are estimated to contribute to one-quarter of all deaths worldwide (Prüss-Ustün et al., 2016). The opioid overdose epidemic in the United States can be seen as a direct consequence of the economic and regulatory structures at play in the country (Hedegaard et al., 2020). Similarly, demographers Case and Deaton have shown that the recent decrease in life expectancy experienced in the country can be partly explained by a rise in "deaths of despair," linked to suicide, alcohol and drug use, and cardiovascular diseases (Case and Deaton, 2015).

3. **Improvement in case fatality rates:** Several changes have occurred in the quantity, distribution, organization and quality of health services that have contributed to the epidemiological transition. Starting mainly during the twentieth century, medical research and technological development have resulted in major advances for the effective management of many diseases, both infectious and non-communicable. An important part of improved survival is due to the decrease of case fatality rates achieved by the application of effective diagnostic and therapeutic technologies.

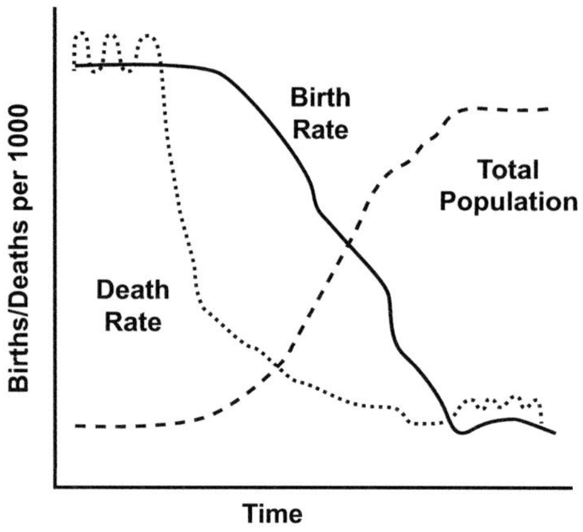

Figure 6.3 Stylized depiction of the demographic transition.

Therapeutic interventions, such as the treatment of pulmonary tuberculosis with specific drugs, acute respiratory infections with antibiotics or acute diarrhea with oral rehydration salts, do not modify the probability of becoming ill, except insofar as early treatment reduces the risk of spreading the disease to others in the population. The main effect of therapeutic interventions is to diminish the probability of death among those who are already ill. In the case of chronic diseases, this type of intervention produces the paradoxical effect of increasing the absolute morbidity level by extending the average duration of the disease (Gruenberg, 1977; Riley, 1990; Rechel et al., 2020). In contrast, primary preventive interventions, such as immunization, do act on the probability of becoming ill. This was evident during the COVID-19 pandemic, where the rapid development and deployment of effective vaccines, coupled with other public health measures like the mandatory use of face coverings, reduced the ability of infected individuals to spread the disease. The main effect of both therapeutic and preventive interventions has been a reduced proportion of deaths caused by infectious diseases, thus contributing to the initial stages of the epidemiological transition. In more advanced stages of the transition, technological innovations may produce a decrease of the case fatality rate or even (although less common) of the incidence of some non-communicable diseases. Together with other factors, this may result in an epidemiological pattern that Olshansky and Ault characterize as the postponement of deaths caused by degenerative diseases (Olshansky and Ault, 1986).

6.3.3 Attributes

The diversity of modalities that each of the three mechanisms may assume in different historical contexts explains why the transition is not a uniform process in every nation or region. Indeed, the characteristics of each mechanism, as well as their interrelationships, establish important differences in the epidemiological dynamics of a country.

First, it is important to establish the basic patterns of change. Beyond its various manifestations, the epidemiological transition always includes three fundamental change processes in the configuration of a population health profile, that is, its patterns of mortality, morbidity and disability. Such changes refer to the composition of cause-specific mortality, the age structure of mortality and the relative weight of morbidity versus mortality in the epidemiological situation.

In the twentieth century, most countries followed a similar epidemiological transition, leading to similar patterns of mortality, morbidity and disability. In the first place, the mortality decline that accompanied the start of the transition was selectively concentrated on infectious diseases, which thereby tend to be displaced by non-communicable diseases, injuries and recognized mental illness. Second, the burden of death and diseases shifted from the younger to the older groups. As we mentioned above, this process was due primarily to two mechanisms: (a) a decline in the incidence and case fatality rates of infectious diseases, which benefited mainly the young population, since infections are more frequent and severe among them; (b) a change in the age structure of the population resulting from the demographic transition, which generated a higher proportion of adults.

The third direction was the change from a health picture dominated by mortality to one where morbidity is the predominant force. Indeed, as mentioned above, the epidemiological transition implies a profound transformation in the social meaning of disease. Instead of being something acute, from which one either recovers or dies, disease becomes a chronic, frequently stigmatizing condition, with increasing psychological, social and economic burdens.

Establishing these basic patterns of change is important to develop a model that can help understand how health conditions evolve and change. Nevertheless, it does not mean that countries will automatically follow this exact pattern. In the following sections, we discuss several limitations of this model.

6.4 Health Transition or Health Transitions?

In his seminal 1971 article, Omran highlights the "classical or Western model" of transition as the standard for comparison. This formulation envisages the epidemiological transition as a progression of ages or stages, from "pestilence and famine" to "receding pandemics" and "degenerative and man-made diseases" (Omran, 1971). This linear and unidirectional view of the transition was shared by other authors. For example, according to Frederiksen (1969), the predominant patterns of morbidity, mortality and fertility, as well as the organization of health care, correspond to four "stages" of society: "traditional," "early transitional," "late transitional" and "modern." Similarly, Lerner (1973) presents three stages, which he calls "low vitality," "increasing control over mortality" and "broadened conception of health." Later authors have proposed additional stages (Rogers and Hackenberg, 1987).

By selecting Western Europe as the standard for comparison, all these authors conformed to a Euro-centric vision of the world. This vision does not adequately reflect the variety and complexity of health transitions around the world.

The usefulness of these stages is limited since they tend to create a linear and unidirectional view of the transition. In reality, several periods or stages may overlap. For instance, the decline of infectious diseases may be slow or even stagnate among important population strata, while non-communicable diseases may be increasing rapidly in another segment of the same population. For example, Defo, using empirical evidence from 57 African countries, showed that many countries experienced different paths from those described by Omran and other authors, leading him to conclude that "prevailing frameworks of demographic, epidemiological and health transitions ... [were] incomplete or irrelevant for charting the population and health experiences and prospects of national populations in the African context" (Defo, 2014).

Furthermore, what has happened, and is still happening in many societies, is that the three basic change patterns described above proceed at different rates among the different social strata and/or regions of a country (Possas, 1989; Marinho et al., 2013). For example, if changes are slower among the poor than the rich, then the former will necessarily have a higher incidence of infectious diseases affecting their larger proportion of young population. An "epidemiological polarization" is thus produced, which worsens health inequalities. This led to the proposal of a "protracted and polarized" transition model to describe the specific situation observed in most middle-income countries and now also in many low-income countries, where an overlap of stages persists over a long period of time and the social distribution of changes is very heterogeneous among social groups (Frenk et al., 1991b).

In any event, it is clear that the dynamics of epidemiological change vary substantially among and within countries. For this reason, and in line with Murray and Chen, it might be more adequate to talk about "health transitions" rather than "the health transition" (Murray and Chen, 1991).

6.4.1 Transitions and Counter-Transitions

It seems incorrect to assume that change must always occur smoothly and in one direction. As Clare Herrick underscores, this simplistic vision perpetuates a "global public health myth" of a world neatly divided between diseases of poverty and diseases of affluence (Herrick, 2022). In addition, this model of the epidemiological transition as a linear process mirrors a broader Cartesian vision of progress and modernity as a positive force in the world, a vision increasingly challenged in the "new climatic regime" we now live in (Latour, 2018).

Rather than the progressive linear trend, a reversal of trends may occur. The most outstanding example is the toll of the HIV/AIDS epidemic, which has claimed millions of lives since the 1980s, and led to important decreases in life expectancy in some countries. Similarly, there may be relapses of infections that had been previously controlled, such as malaria and dengue fever. In other words, small or large "counter-transitions" often take place.

But these counter-transitions may actually be part of the transition itself. There is increased evidence for the bidirectional relationships between infectious and non-communicable diseases. This is one of several false dichotomies that have led to confusion regarding global health priorities (Frenk and Gómez-Dantés, 2017). In the twentieth century, international health was identified with control of infectious diseases, which were supposed to be characteristic of low-income and middle-income countries. Non-communicable diseases, in contrast, were practically absent from the global health agenda, under the belief that they would be limited for quite a long time to high-income countries. In actuality, non-communicable diseases are already the main cause of death and disability in middle-income countries, and their prevalence is rapidly rising in low-income nations (World Health Organization, 2022b). At the other end of the development spectrum, infections never disappeared from wealthy countries, and COVID-19, HIV/AIDS and antibiotic resistance have been strong reminders of the danger of lowering the guard against communicable diseases. In addition, some ailments originally classified as non-communicable have subsequently been found to be linked to an infectious cause. It is estimated that one-fifth of all cancers worldwide are caused by chronic infections produced by agents such as HIV, human papillomavirus (HPV) and hepatitis B virus. Other infections and parasitic diseases are the cause of other non-communicable diseases, such as rheumatic heart disease, Chagas cardiomyopathy and peptic ulcers. Conversely, obesity and pre-existing non-communicable diseases have been linked with a significant increase in the probability of dying from COVID-19 (Katzmarzyk et al., 2020). This means that changes in risk factors for non-communicable diseases could also lead to increased susceptibility to infectious diseases, a theory that could in part help explain the "Africa COVID paradox," which has seen African countries overall experience lower COVID-19 infections and mortality rates than other regions despite higher levels of poverty and severely resource-constrained health systems (Lawal, 2021). In sum, infectious diseases are not the exclusive domain of a "primitive" stage in the health transition, as is often portrayed in the original theories, but rather a shifting component of every epidemiological pattern. Chapter 14 further elaborates on the way COVID-19 has revealed the complex connections between infectious and non-communicable diseases.

As an additional layer of complexity, the stress imposed by human activities on Earth's ecosystems might be further impacting disease incidence by changing transmission patterns for infections. For example, deforestation has been linked with an increase in animal-to-human transmission of zoonotic diseases. The rise of antimicrobial resistance is clearly associated with human and animal overconsumption of antibiotics. The change in risk factors brought about by the social and economic transitions experienced across the globe since the end of World War II might lead to an increase in non-communicable diseases *and* a change in the frequency, severity and distribution of infectious diseases.

Where does this leave us? The change patterns described above are useful to help us understand how health conditions evolve and change. Nevertheless, the epidemiological transition that underpins them, while useful to describe and analyze the megatrends observed in morbidity and morbidity patterns since the twentieth century, is not in itself an archetype easily followed. We observe very different health transitions across countries, socioeconomic groups and periods. At the same time, such patterns should now be supplemented by a more thorough understanding of the relationships between health and the broader environment in a time of rapid ecological change.

The case of neglected tropical diseases (NTDs) outlined in Box 6.1 illustrates both the strengths and limitations of the health transition model. It is essential to understand the mechanisms through which changes in demographics or risk factors affect their prevalence, while also keeping in mind the limits of models for depicting complex, changing realities.

6.4.2 Consequences

The epidemiological transition is ultimately a component of a broader "health transition" (Frenk et al., 1989a). As we posited before, the study of health in populations comprises two major objects: on the one hand, the health conditions of the population; on the other, the social response to those conditions. According to this simplifying

Box 6.1 Neglected tropical diseases: old or new challenge?

The term "neglected tropical diseases" (NTDs) refers to 20 or more diseases grouped by the World Health Organization and other institutions under a single umbrella. While those diseases, ranging from scabies to snakebite, are caused by different pathogens (virus, bacteria, parasites, toxins) and lead to different health conditions, they have been grouped together as a way to raise attention to them, in part because they are most prevalent among impoverished communities and, as a result, often neglected despite affecting 1.4 billion people around the world.

Previous descriptions of the epidemiological transition would classify these diseases as a remnant from a pre-transitional period (in fact, they are sometimes called "diseases of poverty"). Indeed, many of these ailments were prevalent in high-income countries before they were eradicated in the nineteenth and twentieth centuries, thanks to economic development and improvements in water, sanitation and vector control. In the United States, the Rockefeller Foundation's fight against hookworm, which affected up to 40% of the population in the South during the early twentieth century, is a pioneering example of a successful public health program (Elman et al., 2014). Malaria derives its name from the Italian *mala aria* (bad air) and was endemic for centuries in Europe until eliminated in the mid-twentieth century (Boualam et al., 2021).

But stopping there would be too simplistic. In reality, NTDs are a good example of the complexities of the health transition described in this chapter. First, many of them, like tuberculosis and leprosy, are infectious diseases, but they are not acute. To the contrary, they often operate like chronic diseases, progressing slowly, producing long-term pain and disability and generating stigma.

In addition, their role in relationships with other diseases, including non-communicable diseases, is unclear. In fact, some researchers have posited that parasites, such as hookworms, could play a protective role in the development of autoimmune or inflammatory diseases, such as asthma or multiple sclerosis, although more research is needed in this field (Okada et al., 2010; Briggs et al., 2016).

Last, but not least, as the Earth warms due to climate change, diseases currently found primarily in tropical settings, are (re)spreading to other parts of the world, including southern parts of Europe, the United States and China (Hotez, 2016; Ainsworth, 2023; Xu et al., 2024). Hopes of eliminating the most prevalent NTDs by 2030 are increasingly challenged by this new situation.

dichotomy, the health transition may be divided into two main components. The first one is the epidemiological transition, strictly speaking, which is defined as the long-term process of change in the health conditions of a society, including changes in the patterns of disease, disability and death. The second component, which may be called the "health system transition," refers to the change in the patterns of the organized social response to health conditions. Our definitions are consistent with the formulations of other authors, like Lerner and Caldwell, who also conceived of the epidemiological transition as part of a broader health transition.

Of course, the epidemiological transition has (or should have) a profound effect on the health system. The emergence of non-communicable diseases usually aggravates the pressure on complex services. The growing demand for more specialized human resources and more elaborate technologies (which are not necessarily more effective) tends to increase costs. The epidemiological polarization is then more likely to produce a competition for the definition of priorities among diseases and for the corresponding allocation of resources. In order to manage the conflicts that may result, it is necessary to develop innovative service models that use the epidemiological transition as a guide to achieve a corresponding health system transition (Bobadilla et al., 1990). In the future, the juxtaposition of an unfinished agenda of malnutrition, common childhood infections and maternal deaths with chronic diseases and bursts of acute epidemics may force us to re-evaluate how to flexibly allocate and deploy resources across services and interventions. For example, childhood vaccinations dropped dramatically during the COVID-19 pandemic as health systems diverted resources to address the acute emergency (Dalton et al., 2023). It will be important to increase the resilience of health systems to maximize their performance at all times.

As we have noted before, a theoretical framework is crucial for understanding our contemporary health system. But its importance goes well beyond the conceptual. In today's world, we must be able to anticipate and design health systems that can respond to this dynamism. We should use an enhanced understanding of the epidemiological transition as a guide to achieve a corresponding health system transition.

6.5 Summary

In this chapter we have discussed some of the building blocks for a theory of the health transition. These blocks find their foundation in the original formulations of the theory, drawing upon the deep social and economic transformations and the dramatic changes in mortality and morbidity experienced during the twentieth century. But we take them one step further by specifying the concepts, mechanisms, attributes and consequences of the transition and by positioning them in a twenty-first-century world marked by increasing complexity, interdependence and technological innovation.

In Section 3, we turn to the study of health systems as the vehicle for the organized social response to health conditions.

Comprehension and Discussion Questions

1. Provide examples from your own context of the three megatrends described in this chapter.
2. What are the three mechanisms driving the epidemiological transition?
3. What is the difference between the concepts of demographic transition, epidemiological transition and health transition?
4. What are the main limitations of the concept of epidemiological transition described in this chapter?
5. How can the theories and concepts discussed in this chapter help us understand emerging epidemiological trends, such as new infectious diseases, decreases in life expectancy or the aging of the global population?

Papers from Which This Chapter Is Adapted

Frenk, J., BobadillA, J. L., Stern, C., Frejka, T. & Lozano, R. 1991. Elements for a theory of the health transition. *Health Transition Review*, 1, 21–38.

Section

3

Health Systems: The Organized Social Response

Chapter 7

Understanding Complex Systems

Learning Objectives

- Define health systems.
- Distinguish different categories of health services within health systems, including personal, hybrid and population health services.
- Describe the actors and boundaries of a health system, as well as the role of the State.
- Discuss the role of social systems beyond the health system and their impact on health, distinguishing between health systems, systems of health and governance for health.
- Explain the intrinsic and instrumental goals of health systems.
- Identify the functions that health systems perform.

7.1 Introduction

In this chapter, we move to the second object of analysis of public health: the organized social response to health conditions.

There are several conceptual frameworks aiming to capture the essential elements of health systems (Weisz and Harper, 2024). An influential such effort was developed at the World Health Organization (WHO) by Murray and Frenk (2000). To expand our understanding of health systems, this comprehensive framework poses five fundamental questions:

1. What is a health system?
2. What are health systems for?
3. What is the architecture of a health system in terms of its functions?
4. How good is a health system in terms of its performance?
5. How can we relate health system architecture to performance?

For the rest of the chapter, we focus on addressing the first three of these questions, using a significantly expanded and updated version of this framework, while the last two will be addressed in Chapter 9.

7.2 The Importance of Health Systems

Concern about the way in which we confront threats, risks and harms to our health is a central part of the human experience. Every society develops some form of response to disease. For most of history, this response has been limited to the household and carried out by the family nucleus. Alongside the persistent domestic production of care, the twentieth century witnessed the explosive emergence of a differentiated set of institutions with the specialized function of looking after the health of individuals and communities. Modernization, in fact, has been accompanied by a gradual transfer of health responsibilities from family and religious institutions to the professions and the government.

Today, the differentiated set of organizations we call the health system has become a dominant feature of the social fabric in all but the most remote corners of the planet. Health systems currently absorb 11% of the world economy, about 12 trillion US dollars per year – and growing. Of course, there are huge differences in access to these resources. While the United States spends thousands per person per year on health, several countries in sub-Saharan Africa spend less than $40 (World Health Organization, 2021a).

When we speak of the health revolution of the twentieth century, we typically refer to the spectacular decline in mortality and the dramatic shift in the dominant causes of ill health, from infectious to non-infectious diseases, as detailed in Chapter 6. But equally spectacular and equally dramatic has been the rise of health systems, which now permeate all corners of economic activity, dominate political debate, generate cultural interpretations, spur technological innovation, create deep ethical dilemmas and accompany human beings at the most crucial moments of their existence, from birth to death. Furthermore, the COVID-19 pandemic painfully demonstrated how the good or poor performance of health systems, or in this case, its ability to contain diseases, could swiftly destabilize trade, close borders, affect societies and threaten world peace.

In most contemporary societies, health systems simultaneously represent:

- a source of institutional differentiation, taking over functions previously carried out by the individual and the family;
- an expanding set of complex organizations with distinctive authority structures;
- a source of income and employment for millions of professionals, managers and technicians, who function within an elaborate division of labor;
- a channel for mobilizing, exchanging and redistributing large sums of money, both public and private;
- a focus for technological innovation and a prime site where the common citizen comes into personal contact with science (see Chapter 8);
- a vigorous sector of the economy, with important effects on macroeconomic variables such as productivity, inflation, aggregate demand, employment and competitiveness;
- an arena for political struggle among parties, interest groups and social movements;
- a set of cultural meanings for interpreting fundamental aspects of human experience, such as birth and death, pain and suffering, normalcy and deviance;
- a space where many of the key ethical questions of our times are framed and sometimes answered.

This is why it is so important to understand health systems. Yet, despite a growing interest in health system evaluation in the last decades, understanding the performance of health systems remains a continuous challenge.

Like so many other aspects of the global agenda, interest in health systems has gone through cycles of activity and neglect, depending on the dominant winds in the complex process of agenda setting. Around World War II, debate in high-income countries centered on the expansion of social insurance, while the establishment of modern ministries of health and other essential institutions was paramount in low- and middle-income countries, many of which were just achieving independence. At the global level, primary health care occupied center stage in the late 1970s and early 1980s. Health system reform was a topic of continuous debate throughout the 1990s, leading many countries to implement widespread reforms during those decades. In the early 2000s, the accountability pressure represented by the Millennium Development Goals, along with the expanding pluralism that populated the global health scene, fueled a renewed concern for health systems and universal health coverage (Institute for Health Metrics and Evaluation, 2012). At the time of writing this book, in the wake of the COVID-19 emergency, we observe two competing phenomena: on the one hand, a renewed albeit narrow interest in pandemic preparedness and infectious disease prevention and response, fueled by an increased focus on national and global health security; on the other, the recognition that health systems are part of a broader web of social and economic systems, which together need to be retooled and redesigned to address the complex and interrelated challenges of our times, including poverty, climate change, biodiversity loss, geopolitical conflict, population displacement and individual health and well-being.

The increasing interest in health systems is a positive development. This interest is long overdue. Paraphrasing the legendary Professor Vulimiri Ramalingaswami of India, we need more money for health, but we must also deliver more health for the money. There is growing recognition that additional funding can only be effective if national and local health systems are strengthened. In a virtuous circle, better results will be crucial to maintain the momentum of increased funding for health.

7.3 What Is a Health System?

To understand health systems, we first need to ask ourselves what a health system is, drawing upon the WHO framework (World Health Organization, 2000). Many people give up on understanding health systems even before they begin, hindered by three common misconceptions, which present the health system as a black box, a black hole or a laundry list.

The "black box" misconception is the belief that things are too complicated, and we don't know what works, so we simply get technologies and other inputs in place and hope that outputs will somehow work their way. Yet, we have built a sufficient body of knowledge to be able to open the black box and devise specific interventions to improve the performance of the health system. There is a mounting body of evidence on what works and what does not in different settings.

The "black hole" misconception is the common view that no amount of money will suffice to achieve the desired results. As with the dreaded astronomical bodies, health systems absorb enormous amounts of energy, and it is sometimes difficult to find the light in them. Yet, we know that some systems are much more efficient in achieving better results with limited resources.

What we call the "laundry list" view is a sort of "inventory" approach, in which the health system is defined as a mere list of the different organizations or persons that participate in producing health services, without requiring that such components be coordinated or integrated.

Part of the problem with the health systems debate is that too often it has adopted a reductionist perspective that ignores important aspects. Developing a more comprehensive view requires that we expand our understanding of complex systems.

The word "system" has widely differing usages in engineering, informatics, biology, the social sciences, philosophy and common parlance. In the health field, there are two predominant meanings. The first is what we previously called the inventory approach. In this case, the term system refers to a set of elements that are more or less associated by a common function, without specifying the nature of their interrelations.

The second, more rigorous approach could be called "relational." In this case, the definition of system includes not only its component units but also their interrelations. Hence, a system is not just any set of elements, but rather one whose essence is that the whole is different than the sum of its parts. In Rapoport's words, "[A] system is, roughly speaking, a bundle of relationships" (Rapoport, 1968).

It is beyond the scope of this book to examine the philosophical question of whether there is a single underlying theory that can account for all kinds of systems and whether the properties of higher-order (or more aggregate) systems (like societies) can be inferred from the attributes of lower-order systems (like individuals). Clearly, a major difference between biological and social systems is that while the former tend to harmonize functions in search of a common objective (i.e., survival and reproduction), the latter may be fraught with conflict, so that the interests of some constituent units may not be carried forth by the totality of the system.

Such differences notwithstanding, some thinkers emphasize that an essential characteristic of all systems is the presence of a shared aim or set of aims. Thus, Deming has written: "Without an aim, there is no system" (Deming, 1989). Normatively, it can be stated that a shared aim is a key to developing truly integrated health systems. Nevertheless, the precise nature of such an aim may vary among the different actors of the system.

Whatever their respective aims may be, all adaptive systems tend toward complexity, which can be conceived as the boundary between order and chaos (Ruthen, 1993). Complexity derives not only from the internal relations among the components of the system but also from the relations with the external environment.

In the case of the health system, the trend toward increasing complexity has accelerated during the past century. In this relatively short period of time, the social arrangements for dealing with health have been transformed radically. Nowadays, most people come into contact, whether regular or sporadic, with doctors, nurses, technicians, hospitals, clinics, health centers, pharmacies, clinical laboratories, insurance companies, vaccines, drugs, equipment – all the vast and differentiated set of persons, organizations and technologies that specialize in health. A growing proportion of people are born, die and spend considerable periods of their lives in health-related institutions. During the COVID-19 pandemic, people also learned about less visible parts of health systems, such as epidemiologists working on infectious disease surveillance and contact tracing or regulatory bodies in charge of drug and vaccine approval.

Here, we propose a relational view of health systems (Londoño and Frenk, 1997). From this perspective, a health system can be best understood as a set of structural relationships between two major components: a population and a set of specialized institutions. In essence, every health system involves the interaction between a set of providers and a population. Several elements of complexity characterize this interaction.

Many boundaries have been proposed separating the health system from elements outside of it (Terris, 1978; Roemer, 1991; Hsiao, 1992; Frenk, 1994; Chernichovsky, 1995). Some components such as individual health services delivered at clinics are included in all definitions. There is more controversy around components that lie closer to the boundary; for example, are regulations of seatbelt use and their enforcement part of the health system? All boundary definitions are arbitrary, but to assess health system performance, we must propose an operational boundary.

We construct our operational definition by beginning with the concept of a "health action." A health system includes the resources, actors and institutions related to the financing, regulation and provision of health actions. A health action is defined as any set of activities whose **primary intent** is to improve or maintain health. This primary intent criterion leads to a broad definition of the health system. For example, it includes efforts to improve road and vehicle safety, where the primary intent is to reduce traffic accidents, and it also includes personal health services, whether they actually improve health status or not. One major advantage of the primary intent criterion is that it includes in the assessment of health system performance all actors and institutions who see their primary purpose as contributing to health.

7.3.1 Classification of Health Services within Health Systems

An important implication of this broad definition is that a health system encompasses two categories of services: one focused on an **entire community** or **population**, often referred to as "public health services," and another focused on **individual persons**, typically referred to as health care or medical services.

It is common for organizations and researchers to distinguish between those two categories, recognizing their distinct yet interconnected roles in enhancing health outcomes, but also the fact that they have often been kept separate and, to this day, often remain managed by different institutions. For example, the United States has traditionally separated public health activities, mostly managed by federal, state and local institutions, from the provision of medical care, mostly managed by private entities.

We can distinguish among three categories of health action, depending on who receives the services and who benefits from them (see Table 7.1).

1. **Personal health services:** Also called health care services or medical services, personal health services primarily encompass clinical care, addressing individual health needs, such as screenings, general practitioner visits, hospitalization, specialist consultations and emergency services (World Health Organization, 2014a). In a comprehensive perspective of the health care continuum, this set of services spans prevention, diagnosis, treatment, rehabilitation and palliation. The key feature is that each service can only be provided to one specific individual at a time, who directly benefits from it. For example, a person who receives laser surgery to correct their vision will be the

Table 7.1 Categories of health services

Level of provision	Level of benefit	
	Individual	**Population**
Individual	Personal health services	Hybrid health services
		Public health services
Population		Population health services (public goods)

only recipient of the surgery (their eyes are altered) and the only beneficiary (they can read better).

2. **Hybrid health services:** These refer to actions that are provided directly to individuals but benefit a broader segment of the population. Vaccinations are typically included in this category, as are behavioral interventions, such as tobacco cessation counseling and family planning programs. For example, vaccines play a critical role in strengthening immunity against infectious diseases, reducing the incidence and severity of illnesses and enabling herd immunity (when a disease can no longer spread through a population because of high levels of immunity). While vaccines aim to protect the health of entire populations, a community's health relies on its individual members getting vaccinated. In other words, a person who gets, say, a measles vaccine will be the only recipient (the vaccine jab goes into their arm), but the benefit will be double: they will be directly protected from infection, and they will help stop the spread of the virus to others.
3. **Population health services:** Finally, these typically include actions provided at a community or societal level and benefit everyone therein. This category refers to activities addressing broader social and environmental issues affecting populations at large, such as epidemiological risk surveillance, environmental protection, food and water safety, disaster preparedness and response, and mass health education.
   An example of population health services is the regulatory process that led to the banning of toxic lead in gasoline, which was achieved worldwide in 2021. In this case, no one person received the action in particular, but all benefited from it.

Hybrid and population health services are often grouped into one category, referred to as **public health services.**[1] For example, the American Public Health Association emphasizes the difference between health care and public health services, categorizing the former as treating individuals and the latter as addressing populations to prevent sickness and injury (McDonald et al., 2020).

Figure 7.1 further expands this framework by providing a more detailed typology. This starts with the basic recognition of two main categories of health services: personal and public health services. Most personal health services are clinical services along the continuum described earlier (prevention, diagnosis, treatment, rehabilitation and palliation). Similarly, a large part of public health services is what economists call "public goods," which are defined by the fact that their consumption is non-rivalrous (meaning that consumption by one person does not preclude consumption by others) and non-excludable (meaning that no one can be excluded from the benefits that the good generates). We call these public goods population health services, including, as noted above, health promotion, emergency preparedness and response, epidemiological surveillance, environmental health services and collective services like mass education campaigns.

[1] We find here again the same risk of confusion between the concepts of "public health" and "public health services," which we already underlined in Chapter 2 when discussing public health versus population health. As a reminder, we define public health as an interdisciplinary field of both research and practice related to health conditions, as well as health systems, *including* the organization of personal health services, In contrast, public health services are a subcategory of the totality of health services provided by the system.

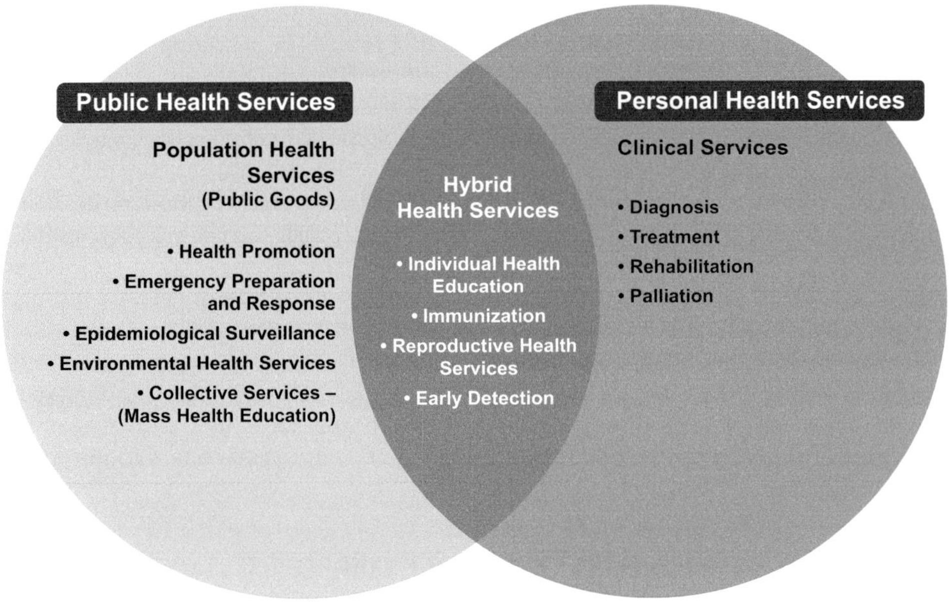

Figure 7.1 Classification of health services.

As shown in Figure 7.1, there is an overlapping category, called hybrid health services, which, as explained earlier, are delivered to individuals but generate benefits for many other members of the community. These benefits are what economists call positive externalities. Compared to public goods, the consumption of hybrid health services is rivalrous, even though the benefits extend to others. Again, vaccines offer a good example. Anyone around vaccinated individuals can experience the benefits, especially when herd immunity is achieved. While many reap the benefit of a vaccinated population, vaccines are prepared as dosages with a limited supply. Therefore, the vaccine dose as a good is rivalrous, since the shot applied to one person is no longer available for another. As can be seen, hybrid health services share attributes of both personal and population health services, which is why we portray them as an overlapping category including services such as individual health education, immunization, reproductive health services and early detection of diseases.

From an institutional perspective, most countries manage population and hybrid services together as the public health subsystem of services. The rest of personal services (i.e., clinical services) are usually managed separately as the health care or medical subsystem.

A common misconception is to equate health systems only with their medical services component, probably because it far outweighs the public health component in terms of volume and resources. Coordinating clinical and public health services is vital for developing a comprehensive health system. In a well-functioning health system, the public health component often provides the broad perspective necessary to identify unmet needs, thereby informing policies and mobilizing resources to support the medical care component. Conversely, medical care is often the first point of contact of patients during an epidemic outbreak and therefore serves to trigger the public health response. One key lesson from the COVID-19 pandemic is the need to better integrate the two subsystems. Indeed, countries with the best records in managing the pandemic had better coordination between medical care and public health services.

It is important to point out that public health professionals straddle both components of the health system. Indeed, while many of them work in public health agencies and community settings, substantial contingents operate within medical care organizations. As a field of practice, the public health workforce brings together multiple professions, such as physicians, nurses, epidemiologists, statisticians, social and behavioral scientists, engineers, managers, lawyers, policy-makers and others. This diverse array of professions underscores the extensive scope of public health work, where efforts are viewed through a population lens aimed at improving the collective well-being of society. Berman and colleagues narrow the broad understanding of public health by breaking it down into manageable components that guide specific characterization of the public health system (Berman et al., 2024). Identifying *what* public health does leads the research team to determine *who* makes up the public health workforce and suggests *how* various actors function together.

7.3.2 Health Systems versus Systems of Health

Notwithstanding the broad definition of health system derived from the primary intent criterion, not all social factors that play a role in determining the health conditions of a population are part of the health system itself. Indeed, many actions that profoundly influence health, such as educating young girls, are not part of the health system, since the primary intent of education is not to improve health. Because it does not meet the primary intent criterion, education should be seen as a determinant of health that lies outside the strictly defined boundaries of the health system.

Such boundaries make sense. They are necessary to assess health system performance and help establish where direct responsibility and stewardship of health actors ultimately lie. A broader definition of health system would be impractical and dilute the meaning of health system per se.

Nevertheless, establishing boundaries does not mean that policies and programs affecting health remain within them. Beyond carrying out health actions in the strict sense, it is necessary to understand how public health actors can address those factors and actions whose primary intent is *not* to improve or maintain health, but which nevertheless have a broad influence on health. Health does not happen in a vacuum. Broader considerations must be taken into account when thinking about how to organize the social response to health conditions. As proposed by Ilona Kickbusch, it is necessary to consider **governance for health**, that is, “the joint actions of health and non-health sectors . . . for a common interest,” alongside **health governance**, that is, the governance and strengthening of the health system itself (World Health Organization, 2014b). Others have discussed the importance of considering **systems of health**, that is, all the systems that relate to health, regardless of whether they belong to the health system or not (McDonald et al., 2020).

This discussion is becoming increasingly relevant in the twenty-first century for two interconnected reasons:

1. **Impact of other systems on health:** As discussed in Chapter 5, the impact of upstream determinants of health is now well documented. A 2020 review by Maani

et al. (2020) identified no less than 48 conceptual frameworks of the determinants of health published since 2000. Evidence abounds on the impact of systemic, societal, institutional, household and individual determinants on health outcomes (World Health Organization, 2021b). In addition, a shift in focus is also taking place. In the last 20 years, discussions on social determinants of health have been primarily framed within the context of health equity. Addressing social determinants was a pathway to deal with persistent health inequalities among vulnerable populations. The COVID-19 pandemic and climate change have demonstrated that focusing on broader determinants of health is essential for achieving health outcomes both for the most vulnerable groups as well as for the entire population, as these complex problems touch upon all sectors of societies and require a much broader response than previously envisioned.

2. **Impact of the health system on other systems:** At the same time, there is a growing recognition of the impact of health actions on other systems. The COVID-19 pandemic has led public actors to recognize how a sub-performing health system could have a catastrophic impact on an entire country's economy, security and well-being. Health is but one of the many challenges faced by modern societies, including poverty, social cohesion, educational attainment, adaptation to and mitigation of climate change, etc. The COVID-19 crisis has laid bare the public policy trade-offs that exist between health and other social benefits. For example, should we prioritize education by reopening schools or prioritize health by closing them? Limit cross-border trade and travel at the expense of economic growth or maintain them? Favor personal choice or impose public health measures? While priority setting across sectors may not be the direct responsibility of health actors, a broader understanding of the synergies and interconnectedness of health and other social goals is essential in today's world.

Environmental determinants offer a good illustration of the "system of health" paradigm. Today, environmental factors are estimated to account for 25% of global deaths (Pruss-Ustun et al., 2016). In addition, the WHO estimates that, between 2030 and 2050, climate change will cause approximately 250,000 additional deaths per year from malnutrition, malaria, diarrhea and heat stress (World Health Organization, 2014b). This could easily counterbalance the positive performance of health systems during that same period. The implications for how health actors operate are enormous. Box 7.1 details one such example, lymphatic filariasis.

Overall, the "rules of the game" are themselves changing as societies and health systems are becoming more fragmented, with power and authority now distributed among multiple actors. Which role precisely should the State play in organizing human activities is increasingly challenged while, at the same time, other actors, including private citizens and commercial organizations, take a more prominent role in shaping health outcomes. And while these other actors may formally belong to health systems according to our definition, the processes and laws to leverage and regulate their participation may not.

We will return to these points later in this chapter when discussing cross-systemic goals, alongside the functions of health systems. At the beginning of this chapter, we concluded that the health system is a set of structured relationships between institutions and populations. Having defined the boundaries of the health system, the next basic question that arises is: Who are the actors that interact within those boundaries?

Box 7.1 Shifting from a health system to a system of health approach to address lymphatic filariasis

Lymphatic filariasis is a neglected tropical disease transmitted through the bites of infected mosquitoes, which has benefited from global coordinated efforts since the launch of the Global Programme to Eliminate Lymphatic Filariasis in 2000. Thanks in large part to the mass drug administration (MDA) of preventive chemotherapy, the number of individuals infected has declined by 74% between 2000 and 2018 (World Health Organization, 2022c). The disease is slated for elimination as a public health problem by 2030. At the same time, climate change is expanding breeding seasons of the mosquitoes responsible for transmitting the disease due to a hotter climate. As Blum and Hotez describe, we are now facing "a race between MDA and climate change-induced expansion of vector ranges" (Blum and Hotez, 2018). Public health professionals need to consider these broader factors and likely collaborate with meteorologists and environmental scientists if they want to succeed in controlling lymphatic filariasis in the long term.

7.3.3 Actors and Relationships

Figure 7.2 presents a simplified view of the main actors operating in the health system. It is common to think of health systems only in terms of the institutions whose primary intent is to improve health. However, a relational view of health systems makes it clear that the population is not an external beneficiary of the system; it is an essential part of it. This is because, when it comes to health, people play five different roles:

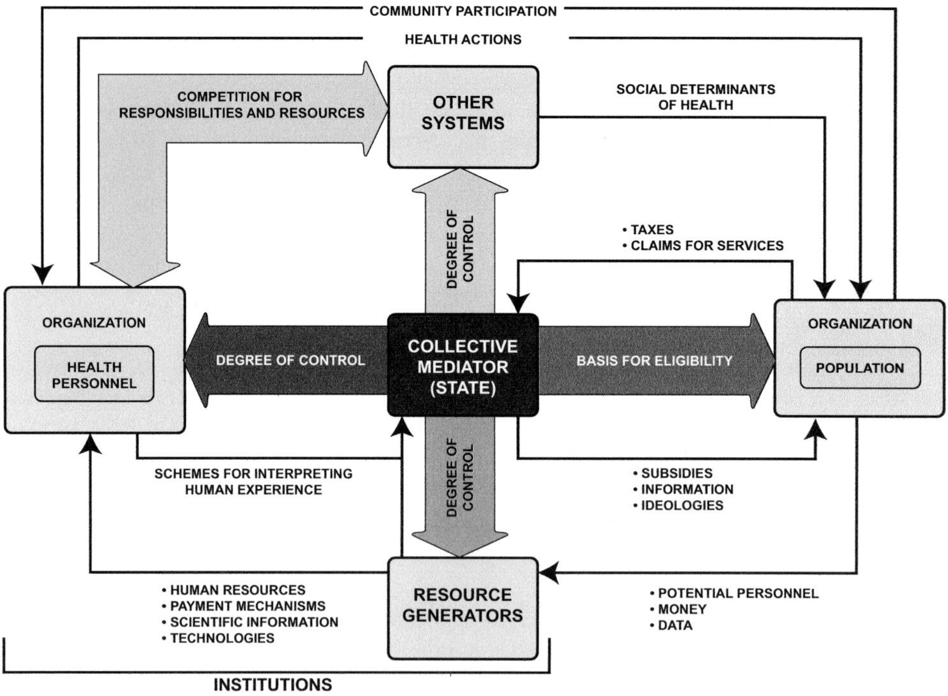

Figure 7.2 Actors and relationships in health systems.

- certainly, as patients, with specific needs requiring care, which is the most common role that we tend to analyze;
- also, as consumers, with specific expectations about the way in which they will be treated;
- as taxpayers and therefore as the ultimate source of financing;
- as citizens who may demand access to care as a right;
- most importantly, as co-producers of health through care seeking, adherence to medications and behaviors that may promote or harm one's own health or the health of others.

This last role was made obvious during the COVID-19 pandemic, when adherence with health recommendations, such as regular handwashing, social distancing, isolation and vaccination were key to controlling the disease.

In these various roles, members of the population interact with health personnel working in institutions. This interaction has several characteristics. First, neither health personnel nor members of the population act in isolation; instead, they belong to various organizations that shape their interaction. The personnel organizations include both their workplaces and the associations representing their interests. In the case of the population, there are several levels of organization, including the household, the community and the many instances in which people are brought together, such as firms, trade unions, political parties, interest groups, etc.

Second, neither personnel nor populations constitute homogeneous categories. Health organizations encompass a wide variety of professional and occupational groups, with different degrees of dominance in the division of labor (Freidson, 2017). There may even be cleavages within a group, such as physicians (Hafferty, 1988). Hence, all personnel do not necessarily share the same interests. In turn, populations are stratified along several lines, of which occupation, income, education, gender, race and geographic location, among others, have very important effects on the distribution of health conditions and on access to providers.

Third, the relationship between personnel and population is not direct, but is mediated by some collective actor (Johnson, 1972). While in the past, such an intermediary role might have been played by religious or other social institutions, in most contemporary countries, the State has become the key collective mediator.[2] As we will see when we discuss the functions of health systems, the degree of control the State exercises depends on how many of those functions it carries out. The normative issue of the appropriate functions to be carried out by the State lies at the heart of the debate on the public/private mix (Frenk, 1993b).

This debate is also directly relevant to the relationship of the State with the population and its organizations. As shown in Figure 7.2, such a relationship rests on the principles established to define the eligibility of different groups to health services. Historically, it is possible to identify four principles: **purchasing power**, which considers health as just one more element of the market economy; **poverty**, which has been the

[2] In this book, we follow the common practice of adopting the narrow definition of the State as the institutions of government providing the administrative, legislative and judicial vehicles for the actual exercise of public authority and power, rather than the broad definition of the State as the total political organization of a society, including its citizens.

basis of public assistance through which the State provides certain services to those who do not have the means to obtain them; **socially perceived priority**, which has found its expression in the social security systems that allow certain strategic groups, such as industrial workers, civil servants or the armed forces, to make financial contributions entitling them to health services and other benefits; and **citizenship**, which implies universal access based on the definition of health as a social right (Soberon et al., 1986). Unfortunately, a lot of the public/private debate has looked only at the pragmatic aspects of policy alternatives. Each of them, however, reflects the values that underlie the foregoing principles. Health system reform projects would be enriched if they made explicit their choice of eligibility principles and then derived the implications for policy design.

As indicated earlier, the population, the personnel and the collective mediator are the central components of health systems. Their interaction is further complicated by the presence of other actors. Thus, they are supported by various organizations that obtain potential resources from the population and transform them into effective health-related resources (Figure 7.2). Such organizations include universities, in the case of human resources and scientific research; insurance firms or social security funds, in the case of financial resources; and the many companies producing technologies. Here, we understand technology in a broad sense: it can include medicines, diagnostics and medical equipment, but also increasingly software or digital technologies focused on health. As in the case of health personnel, the State may exercise varying degrees of control over these resource generators.

Finally, there are many other economic sectors that produce goods and services affecting health (e.g., food, education, housing, water and sanitation, environmental protection). As discussed earlier, many of those sectors are not strictly part of the health system but of the social determinants of health. We include them in the figure because of their crucial interactions with both the health institutions and the population.

7.4 What Are Health Systems for?

Organized activity of society can be divided into various systems, such as health, education, production of consumer goods, politics, culture, security, etc. For each of these systems there is a defining goal, the reason for which the system exists. For the education system, this goal is to educate individuals and for the health system it is to improve health, both the average level and its distribution across individuals. Similarly, the political system's main goal in democracies centers on democratic participation, while a cultural system may focus on the development of knowledge and culture. In addition to the defining goal for each system of society, there are two goals common to all systems: the responsiveness of the system to the legitimate expectations of the population and the fairness in the financial contribution required to make the system work.

For all systems and defining goals, the population will have expectations for how institutions and actors that attempt to achieve that goal interact with them. For example, are human rights respected? What is the degree of autonomous involvement of the individual in decisions? Are people treated with dignity? Likewise, for every system, we have a goal of fairness in financial contribution. What is considered to be fair in this respect may vary considerably for different systems. Perhaps the market mechanism, where what you pay for is what you get, is appropriate for most consumption goods, but for health, education, security and some other systems, the concept of fairness in financial contribution may be very different.

In addition to the intrinsic goals of each system, each system may contribute to several social goals. In other words, the health, education or security systems may and most likely do affect (positively or negatively) the attainment of the defining goals of other systems. Recognizing these interactions, we can define a series of cross-system goals for each system.

For example, health can be both a goal with intrinsic value, as well as an instrumental goal for the attainment of other social goals: how much the health system helps or hinders education, democratic participation, economic production, etc. These cross-system goals are potentially very important and should be the subject of special analysis and evaluation. One of the most important cross-system goals that should be emphasized is the contribution of the health system to economic production. Health and health systems may strengthen or weaken economic growth. For example, some methods of organizing health financing, such as some forms of employment-based insurance, may hinder labor mobility and macroeconomic performance (Gruber and Madrian, 1994; Buchmueller and Valletta, 1999). At the same time, there is increasing evidence that improvements in health can enhance economic growth (Sacks and Gallup, 1999; Bhargava et al., 2001). The COVID-19 pandemic has offered the clearest example of the impact of health on the economy. Indeed, a public health crisis like the pandemic triggered a deep economic crisis throughout the world. This experience has provided further demonstration of the notion that health is not only a consequence but also a determinant of economic development.

7.4.1 Health System Goals

As discussed in Section 7.3, we can more explicitly formulate the three main goals for the health system: health improvement, responsiveness and fair financing. These three intrinsic goals should be routinely monitored by all countries and should form the main basis for the assessment of health system performance. Therefore, the work on operationalizing the measurement of goal attainment is focused on measuring these three goals as well as relating goal attainment to resource use in order to evaluate performance.

The following discussion aims to articulate more precisely the content of each of the three goals.

7.4.1.1 Health Improvement

The defining goal for the health system is to improve the health of the population. If health systems did not contribute to improved health, we would choose not to have them. The health of the population should reflect the health of individuals throughout the life course and include both premature mortality and non-fatal health outcomes as key components. We are concerned both with the average level of population health and with the distribution of health within the population, namely, health inequalities, as already discussed in Chapter 5.

7.4.1.2 Responsiveness

The second intrinsic goal is to enhance the responsiveness of the health system to the legitimate expectations of the population. The term "legitimate" is used to recognize that some individuals may have frivolous expectations for the health system, which should not form part of the articulation of this goal.

We propose that responsiveness has two major components. The first can be called "respect for persons," and it captures aspects of the interaction of individuals with the health system that often have an important ethical dimension. The second component can be called "client orientation," and it includes several dimensions of consumer satisfaction that are not a function of health improvement.

In turn, respect for persons comprises the following three aspects:

1. **Respect for dignity:** Health systems might be able to achieve higher levels of health by incarcerating individuals with a communicable disease or sterilizing individuals with a genetic disorder, but this would be a violation of basic human rights (Muller, 1985; Leavitt, 1995; Pernick, 1997). Respect for dignity also includes aspects of the interaction with providers such as courtesy and sensitivity to potentially embarrassing moments of clinical interrogation or physical exploration (Smith, 1981; World Medical Association, 1981; Brock, 1993; Wainwright, 1994; World Health Organization, 1994; Hendriks, 1997).
2. **Respect the individual's autonomy:** Individuals, when competent, or their agents, should have the right to choose what interventions they do and do not receive (World Health Organization, 1994).
3. **Respect for confidentiality:** In interacting with the health system, individuals should have the right to preserve the confidentiality of their personal health information (Bok, 1986; Beauchamp and Childress, 1989). Respect for confidentiality serves an instrumental goal of improving the quality of health care; when individuals have confidence that the confidentiality of their personal health information will be respected, they are more likely to give important medical history information to health care providers when asked. In addition, respect of confidentiality is intrinsically valuable because it upholds a core notion of privacy and individual control over personal information (Rachels, 1975; Reiman, 1976; Schoeman, 1992; Wainwright, 1994; Sitzia and Wood, 1997; Lowe and Hardy Havens, 1998).

The second component of responsiveness, client orientation, includes several dimensions of consumer satisfaction that are not a function of health improvement. Client orientation comprises the following four aspects:

1. **Prompt attention to health needs:** Surveys of population satisfaction with health services routinely demonstrate that prompt attention is a key dimension (Carr-Hill, 1992; Ross et al., 1995; Thompson and Sunol, 1995; Cohen et al., 1996, Bernhart et al., 1999). Individuals value prompt attention because it may lead to better health outcomes; this value is captured in the defining goal of health. Individuals may also value prompt attention because it can allay fears and concerns that come with waiting for a diagnosis or treatment. The intrinsic value of prompt attention is critically affected by factors such as physical, social and financial access.
2. **Basic amenities:** The basic amenities of health services such as clean waiting rooms or adequate beds and food in hospitals are aspects of care that are often highly valued by the population (Gilson et al., 1994).
3. **Access to social support networks for individuals receiving care:** Even when care is promptly available, if it is provided far from the individual's family and community,

access to social support networks during care and recovery may be hampered (Murray et al., 2013).

4. **Choice of institution and individual providing care:** Patients may want to select who provides them with health care (Cohen et al., 1996). This concern is most often for the individual provider and only secondarily for the institution providing care. Choice is a legitimate component of responsiveness and takes on increasing importance as other items in this list have been satisfied.

As with health, we are concerned not only with the average level of responsiveness but also with inequalities in its distribution. A concern for the distribution of responsiveness across individuals means that we are implicitly interested in differences related to social, economic, demographic and other factors.

7.4.1.3 Fair Financing

To be fair, financing of the health system should address two key challenges. First, households should not become impoverished or pay an excessive share of their income in obtaining needed health care. In other words, fairness in financial contribution requires an important degree of financial risk pooling. Second, poor households should pay less toward the health system than rich households. Not only do poor households have lower incomes, but a larger share of their income goes to basic needs such as food or shelter. Contribution to the health system should reflect this difference in disposable income between those with more or less wealth.

These considerations translate into the normative proposition that every household should pay a fair share of the costs of the health system. (In the case of very low-income households, "fair share" might mean no payment at all.) Payment should be based on income and should mostly not reflect use of services or risk. Sustainability of health financing may benefit from a broad acceptance of social solidarity in financing, which requires everyone to contribute some fair share.

In attempting to summarize our view of health system goals, Table 7.2 shows that we are interested in the level and distribution of health improvement and responsiveness, but only in the *distribution* of the financing burden, not in the absolute level of financing of the health system. The average level of financing is not an intrinsic goal for the health system. Rather, the level of health financing is one of the key policy choices for society. The level of resources invested in the health system is the variable against which goal attainment is compared in order to measure performance. In the sections that follow we stress the prominence of resources available for the health system as the critical comparator to goal attainment. The level of goal attainment for health and responsiveness

Table 7.2 Health system goals

	Level	Distribution	
Health improvement	✓	✓	Efficiency
Responsiveness	✓	✓	
Fair financing	X	✓	
	Quality	Equity	

can be considered as the overall quality of the health system. This is a broader concept than definitions of quality focused on personal health services alone (Donabedian, 1980; Daniels et al., 1996). As explained more fully below, quality is a subset of overall goal attainment, not a performance measure.

The fairness of the distributions of health, responsiveness and financial burden are the key components of the equity of the health system. As with quality, equity of the health system is a subset of overall goal attainment and not a performance measure. Our conception of the equity of the health system is broader than simply health inequalities, since it also includes unequal responsiveness to different social groups (Bok, 1995).

A third related concept is efficiency or composite goal performance. Efficiency is how well the level and distribution of the three main goals for the health system are achieved compared to the available resources. Societies will inevitably differ on the weights that they attach to the five components (checks) shown in Table 7.2. In 2000, the *World Health Report* proposed a ranking of the health systems of its 191 member states based on a composite measure of health system goal attainment, building upon an earlier version of the framework presented in this chapter (World Health Organization, 2000). While the ranking itself was not continued in subsequent years, the report sparked increased attention to the performance of health systems and the factors explaining such performance.

7.4.1.4 Instrumental Goals

Absent from our parsimonious list of three main goals for health systems are many that have been prominently featured in discussions of health system performance, such as access to care, community involvement, innovation or sustainability. While we do not doubt their importance, these are instrumental goals whose attainment will raise the level of attainment of health, responsiveness and fairness in financing. For example, consider the goal of access to care. Improved access to care is desirable only insofar as it improves health, reduces health inequalities and enhances responsiveness. Access to care is an important instrumental albeit not intrinsic goal for health systems. If measurement of the attainment of the three intrinsic goals is done adequately, we will fully reflect the impact of access to care and other instrumental goals on the outcomes that are valued by society. Likewise, coverage of many effective public health programs, such as directly observed therapy for tuberculosis, immunization or impregnated bed-nets for malaria, are instrumental goals that would be captured in the measurement of health and responsiveness.

7.5 What Is the Architecture of a Health System in Terms of Its Functions?

In every health system, organizations must perform five basic functions: financing, provision, resource generation (human, physical and knowledge), stewardship and systemic integration, as shown in Figure 7.3. Every health system grapples with the key problems of designing, implementing, evaluating and reforming the institutions that perform or facilitate these functions. It is possible to compare such solutions along three major categories, which form a continuum going from broad policy directions to specific operational attributes: **strategic design**, **structural arrangements** and **implementation management**. In the following sections, we specify the elements for each function. Of note, those functions apply both to personal health services and public health services,

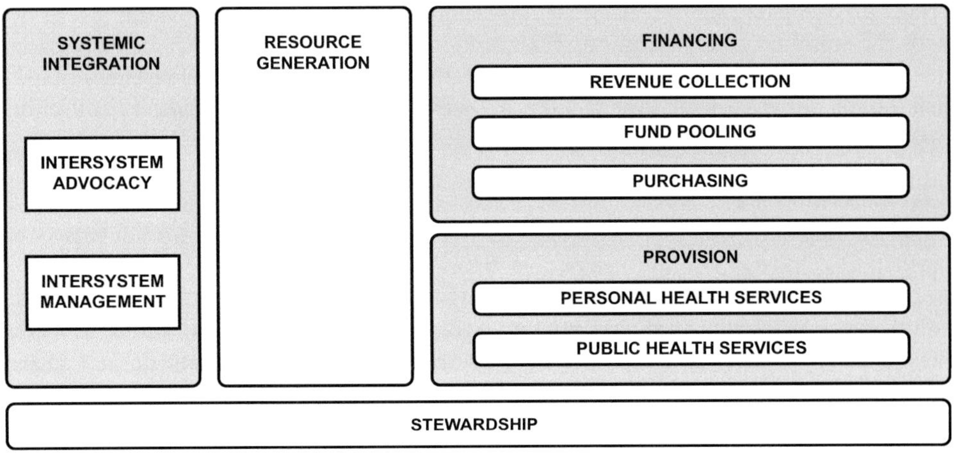

Figure 7.3 Functions of health systems. Adapted from *Bulletin of the World Health Organization*, Vol. 78, No. 6, Murray, C. J. & Frenk, J., "A framework for assessing the performance of health systems," pages 717–731. Copyright (2000).

as defined earlier. The strategic design, structural arrangements and implementation management of each function will likely include a mix of options to accommodate the specificities of each type of service.

7.5.1 Financing

Health system financing is the process by which revenues are collected from primary and secondary sources, accumulated in fund pools and allocated to specific activities of particular providers. For the purposes of analysis, it is useful to subdivide health system financing into three subfunctions: revenue collection, fund pooling and purchasing.

7.5.1.1 Revenue Collection

Revenue collection refers to the mobilization of money from primary sources (households and firms) and secondary sources (governments and donor agencies). Funds can be mobilized through eight basic mechanisms: out-of-pocket payments, voluntary insurance rated by income, voluntary insurance rated by risk, compulsory insurance, general taxes, earmarked taxes, donations from non-governmental organizations and transfers from donor agencies.

The strategic design of revenue collection is likely to profoundly affect health system performance. Some of the key dilemmas that decision-makers face include compulsory versus voluntary payments, prepayment versus payment at the point of service and progressivity of insurance premiums, fees or taxes. Particular to this debate is how those criteria are selected for different services. For example, tobacco or alcohol taxes are typically earmarked for public health services, while the provision of personal health services may come from a combination of taxation, insurance and out-of-pocket payments. Research and development activities, such as vaccine development can benefit from government contributions, but also investments from private firms. In terms of the structural arrangements of revenue collection, a key aspect with potential effects on performance is the governance of institutions, mostly as it refers to the extent of public versus private participation. Another important matter for decision-making has to do with the number of organizations that carry out this function, which in turn raises questions of economies of scale and concentration. Implementation management issues that might affect performance include measures to avoid evasion, specific collection procedures and earmarking of taxes.

7.5.1.2 Fund Pooling

Fund pooling refers to the accumulation of revenues for the common advantage of participants. Indeed, pooling means that financial resources in the pool are no longer tied to a particular contributor. In the language of insurance, pooling means that contributors share financial risk. Pooling is distinct from revenue collection, as some mechanisms of revenue collection such as medical savings accounts do not share financial risks across contributors (Frenk et al., 1989b).

Aspects of the strategic design of fund pooling likely to affect performance include the extent to which there are separate fund pools for different population groups, separate fund pools for personal and public health services and cross-subsidization between low- and high-risk contributors. Structural arrangements of fund pooling include the size and number of fund pools, mechanisms to transfer funds among pools, choice and competition among fund pools for enrollment and governance of institutions maintaining fund pools. A critical implementation management question that might affect performance refers to rules that guide the entry and exit of organizations performing this function, including procedures for protecting contributors in the case of insolvency or bankruptcy. Another regulatory matter has to do with the rules governing the financial management of funds, including the degree of investment risk that is allowed.

7.5.1.3 Purchasing

Purchasing is the process through which revenues that have been collected and placed in fund pools are allocated to institutional or individual providers in order to deliver a specified or unspecified set of interventions. Purchasing can range from simple budgeting exercises in highly integrated public systems, where the government collects revenue through general taxation and allocates it to programs and facilities for staff and other costs, to more complicated strategies where specified units of inputs, outputs or outcomes are purchased.

Strategic design includes decisions on what is purchased, how it is purchased and from whom it is purchased. Choosing what is purchased has to do with the implicit or explicit criteria used to select interventions for inclusion or exclusion. Alternative mechanisms include direct purchasing of interventions (coronary artery bypass grafts, childhood immunizations, etc.), more general purchasing of service types (physician services, hospital bed-days, etc.) or purchasing of inputs (doctors, hospital beds or vehicles). Another aspect of strategic design is the choice of providers to deliver interventions, including issues such as command-and-control procedures or contractual processes that relate the purchaser to providers, the criteria for choosing providers and provider payment mechanisms.

Structural arrangements that may affect performance include the size and number of purchasers, mechanism of funding from revenue pools to purchasers, choice and competition between purchasers for enrollment and governance of purchasers. The most important implementation management matters refer to the methods for controlling the quantity and the quality of purchased services. It is beyond the scope of this book to examine the vast array of utilization review and quality assurance techniques that may be used to orient purchasing decisions. Many of them form the core of what has been termed "managed care."

7.5.2 Provision of Health Services

This function refers to the combination of inputs into a production process that takes place in a particular organizational setting and that leads to the delivery of a series of interventions. In analyzing provision, it is useful to keep in mind the distinction between personal and public health services, as discussed earlier. The former refer to services that are consumed directly by an individual, whether they are preventive, diagnostic, therapeutic, rehabilitative or palliative, and whether they generate externalities or not. Public health services refer to actions applied either to whole populations (e.g., mass health education) or to the non-human components of the environment (e.g., basic sanitation).

7.5.2.1 Personal Health Services

The strategic design of the provision of personal health services deals mostly with the relationships of each provider organization to its environment. One set of such relationships has to do with vertical integration among functions. While this matter is analyzed in more general terms below, it is necessary to underscore its importance for the provision function, since in this case the most fundamental design question refers to the extent of integration with the purchasing function. Indeed, national health systems are often distinguished according to whether these two functions are carried out by the same organization or whether providers are independent contractors for purchasing entities. One of the main policy proposals for integrated systems is precisely the "purchaser–provider split." Closely linked to this matter is the issue of decentralization and governance of provider institutions, particularly with respect to the extent of autonomy even in a framework of public ownership. The extent to which such fundamental design options affect the performance of health systems is an important research question with major policy implications.

Structural arrangements have to do mostly with the relationships of provider organizations to each other. A central question is the extent to which such organizations are separate entities or whether they form networks at different levels of complexity (i.e., primary, secondary and tertiary health care facilities). The structure of such networks will determine whether access to a facility is direct or whether there is a gatekeeping role for first-contact providers. This is one instance of the more general problem of organizing referrals among levels of care, including whether referrals can cross public–private boundaries or whether private and public networks are segregated from each other.

In contrast to the first two aspects of provision, issues related to implementation management have to do mostly with the internal dimension of each provider organization including an understanding of both the formal and the informal ways in which each organization articulates its tasks, control systems and relationships of authority. Staffing patterns for both management and clinical services are important elements (World Bank, 1987). Typical issues include whether top management of provider organizations is in the hands of physicians or professional administrators. At the clinical level, the question of skill mix among the various categories of providers (physicians, nurses, community health workers, etc.) is also likely to be a determinant of performance.

7.5.2.2 Public Health Services

Conceptually, the same categories of issues apply to public health as to personal health services. Nevertheless, in most countries local and national governments take a dominant role in the provision of public health services. A key question in terms of strategic design is the extent to which single organizations provide a wide array of public health services or multiple specialist organizations provide specific services such as health promotion, occupational safety, road traffic safety or infectious diseases surveillance. As with personal health services, the extent of integration with purchasing is important, as is the nature of governance and autonomy.

In terms of structural arrangements, a main issue appears to be the degree of integration of the provision of public health with personal health services. In public systems, are the same organizations and managers responsible for both categories of services? In systems with private providers of personal health services, are there incentives and other mechanisms for them to also deliver some public health services, like mass health education?

Finally, the same issues of intra-organizational management that were highlighted for the provision of personal health services would apply here as well.

7.5.3 Resource Generation

Health systems are not limited to the set of institutions that finance or provide services but include a diverse group of organizations that produce inputs to those services, particularly human resources, physical resources, such as facilities and equipment, and knowledge. This set of organizations encompasses universities and other educational institutions, research centers and the vast array of organizations producing specific technologies such as pharmaceutical products, devices and equipment.

Questions of strategic design, structural arrangements and implementation management will vary according to the specific subset of organizations involved in resource generation. For example, in the case of educational institutions such as medical and nursing schools, a key issue refers to their primary organizational location, whether they belong to the ministry of health or the ministry of education. Organizational ownership may determine the match between the supply of and the demand for health personnel. In the case of research organizations, questions of autonomy in determining priorities become salient. In the case of the pharmaceutical and other technological industries, common questions of industrial structure, such as the degree of concentration and the extent of competition, are very likely to influence health system performance.

7.5.3.1 Focus: Human Resources for Health

Professionals, technicians and other workers represent the indispensable resource for health systems. The reason is simple: health is all about people. The core space of every health system is occupied by the unique encounter between one set of people who need services and another who have been entrusted to deliver them. This trust is earned through a special blend of technical competence and service orientation, steered by ethical commitment and social accountability, which forms the core of professional work. Developing such a blend requires a prolonged period of education and a substantial investment on the part of both student and society.

In Chapter 6, we reviewed the dramatic health revolution that led to a doubling of life expectancy during the twentieth century. Arguably, dramatic reforms in the education of health professionals helped to catalyze last century's health gains. Coming on the heels of the discovery of germ theory in Europe, the opening of the twentieth century witnessed widespread reforms in professional education around the world. In the United States, such reports as by Flexner (1910), Welch and Rose (1915) and the Committee for the Study of Nursing Education and Goldmark (1923) transformed post-secondary education of physicians, public health workers and nurses, respectively. These efforts to embed a scientific foundation into the education of health professionals significantly transformed the fields of public health and medicine.

Yet, most health systems in the world are beset by difficult challenges related to their workforce, including major imbalances in the number, competency and geographic distribution of health professionals. At the same time, educational institutions struggle to meet the demands of health systems and the needs of the population. On the bright side, there are now instructional and institutional innovations that may usher in a new era in the development and deployment of the health workforce. The COVID-19 pandemic accelerated the adoption of many of those innovations.

To mark the centennial of the Flexner report, the journal *The Lancet* convened the Commission on the Education of Health Professionals for the 21st Century. Published in 2010, its report offered a detailed diagnosis, along with a series of reform proposals, many of which have been implemented around the world (Frenk et al., 2010). To take stock of the many changes that took place in the decade after the publication of this report and of the impact of the COVID-19 pandemic on the education of health professionals, *The Lancet* published an update in 2022 (Frenk et al., 2022).

7.5.4 Stewardship

A neglected function in most health systems, stewardship goes beyond the conventional notion of regulation. It involves three key aspects: setting, implementing and monitoring the rules of the game for the health system; assuring a level playing field among all actors in the system (particularly purchasers, providers and patients); and defining strategic directions for the health system as a whole. In order to deal with these aspects, stewardship can be subdivided into five subfunctions: overall system design, performance assessment, priority setting, regulation and consumer protection.

Overall system design has to do with policy formulation at the broadest level. It involves the way in which all the other health system functions are put together. The various issues that have been analyzed above under the rubric of strategic design form the substantive content for this subfunction of stewardship. In this respect, stewardship can be thought of as a "meta-function," insofar as it deals with the organization of all the other functions of a health system.

An essential ingredient to provide strategic direction and assure a level playing field is to assess the performance of institutions involved in revenue collection, purchasing, provision and resource generation. This is another meta-function.

Designing criteria for setting priorities and conducting a consensus-building process around them are major elements of stewardship. This involves both a technical and a political aspect.

Strictly speaking, regulation means setting rules of the game. In the health system, there are two main types: sanitary regulation of goods and services and health care regulation. The former refers to the conventional efforts by sanitary authorities to minimize the health hazards that might be generated by the goods and services provided throughout the economy, especially those that are directly consumed by human beings, such as food or beverages. The latter is applied to organizations charged with the financial, provision and resource generation functions of the health system. In this respect, regulation is again a meta-function directed to institutions charged with other functions, through instruments such as accreditation, certification, rate setting and others.

Both the insurance and the health care markets are characterized by information and power asymmetries between consumers and producers. Therefore, achieving a level playing field among the actors of the health system requires explicit efforts at consumer protection as part of the stewardship function.

The mix of these five subfunctions of stewardship is the key decision regarding its strategic design. Indeed, there seems to be remarkable variation in the extent to which health authorities assume responsibility for each subfunction.

With respect to structural arrangements, the main policy consideration refers to the locus of responsibility. While stewardship generally entails a set of core public functions, there is variation on the allocation of responsibility to different branches (executive versus legislative) and levels (national versus local) of government.

Finally, an important question of implementation management affecting performance refers to the actual skills to carry out stewardship functions. In particular, the reorientation of most ministries of health from their traditional function as providers of services to the new challenges of stewardship involves major organizational re-engineering for which the skill mix may not be adequate.

7.5.5 Systemic Integration

Finally, health systems carry out a fifth function,[3] primarily focused on the relationships between the health system and other social systems. This function can be divided into two subfunctions: intersystem advocacy and intersystem management.

Intersystem advocacy aims to influence the way non-health sectors impact health goals, both to address the negative impact and harness the positive impact of actions outside the health system. It builds upon a long tradition of health promotion, historically centered on health education and individual behavior, which has evolved in recent decades to adapt them to our modern, interconnected societies. In particular, it borrows from two interrelated concepts: first, the Healthy Public Policy, introduced by Nancy Milio in the 1980s, which emphasizes the need to more explicitly consider health and equity in all areas of policy beyond the health sector and therefore the need to create accountability mechanisms to ensure health impact (Milio, 1981); second, the Health in All Policies framework, developed by the WHO since the 1980s, which promotes the idea that non-health processes should be adapted to incorporate public health aspects, even

[3] Of note, this fifth function was not included in the previous iteration of the framework published by Murray and Frenk (2000), but is a new addition, based on recent evolutions in health systems and societies in general.

for areas that do not directly collaborate with the health sector but nevertheless impact health outcomes (Stahl et al., 2006). Health impact assessments, for example, inspired by environmental health impact assessments, have been developed as a tool to better understand the health impact of policies and programs from other sectors. In some countries, public health coordinators have been placed within local authorities to ensure health is systematically considered in all policies (Hagen et al., 2018a).

Intersystem management incorporates within the scope of health systems the responsibility to manage the impact of health systems on other systems. This function posits that health system actors should influence public policy decisions to ensure health system goals are correctly assessed and selected against other social goals, and to consider the role that health may play as an intrinsic goal in the impact pathway of other social goals. Building upon our earlier discussion on cross-system goals, intersystem management attempts to articulate the role that health plays in other systems.

At its simplest, the subfunction of intersystem advocacy treats health as the outcome of actions in multiple systems whereas intersystem management treats health as the determinant of effects on other systems.

Aspects of the strategic design of systemic integration include the roles and responsibilities of different public and private actors to achieve such integration, as well as how the pathways and connections between health and non-health goals are understood by the different actors. Structural arrangements of systemic integration include the way in which budget and management processes, both within governments and with other actors, can lead to such integration across systems. Finally, an important question of implementation management refers to the question of how to design the roles and responsibilities and incentivize health and non-health actors to perform actions beyond their traditional scope of activities or interests.

7.6 Summary

In this chapter, we have addressed three key questions about health systems: What is a health system? What are health systems for? And what functions should a health system perform? In summary, a health system can be best understood as an interconnected set of structural relationships between two major components: a population and a set of providers. A health system includes the resources, actors and institutions related to the financing, regulation and provision of activities, whose primary intent is to improve or maintain health. Health systems include personal health services (e.g., medical visits), hybrid health services (e.g., vaccination) and population health services (e.g., water safety), the combination of the latter two often described as public health services.

Health systems are different from systems of health, which include all the systems that relate to health, and governance for health, which is interested in the broader actions and systems involved in achieving health outcomes. Usually, the relationship between providers and population is not direct, but is mediated by some collective actor, which is usually the State. The State can participate in health through three major mechanisms: regulation, financing and direct delivery of services.

The defining purpose of the health system is to improve health, both the average level and its distribution across individuals. Two other important intrinsic goals of the health system should be responsiveness to the legitimate expectations of the population and fairness in the financial contribution required to make the system work.

Health systems must perform five basic functions: financing (revenue collection, fund pooling and purchasing), provision, resource generation (human, physical and knowledge), stewardship and systemic integration. Those functions apply to personal, hybrid and public health services, albeit with slight differences across categories.

Having covered the basic concepts of health systems, we turn our attention to one key aspect of health systems: health technologies.

Comprehension and Discussion Questions

- Consider the definition of a health system. With this definition, are advocacy groups focused on climate change part of the health system? What about lawyers and pharmaceutical companies?
- What is the difference between a health system and a health care system?
- What are the benefits of a broad health system definition? What are the risks?
- We discussed Health in All Policies. How does this approach compare with the definition of a health system based on "primary intent" to improve or maintain health?
- If an activity is defined as part of the health system, does it mean it should be under the authority of the ministry of health? Why or why not?
- We include the population as part of the health system. Do you think this is important? Why?
- What is the difference between intrinsic and instrumental goals?
- We identify three separate intrinsic goals for a health system. But one could say health is the only goal of a health system. What are the implications of this statement? Provide an example.
- Is the level of health financing important for a health system? Why or why not?
- Who assesses if expectations of the population are legitimate?
- Can you think of situations when these different goals were (or were not) realized during the COVID-19 crisis?
- The WHO includes "improved efficiency" as an explicit goal of health systems. Do you think it matters? Why or why not?
- Do you think the mix of public and private actors is important for a health system. Why or why not?

Papers from Which This Chapter Is Adapted

Frenk, J. 1994. Dimensions of health system reform. *Health Policy*, 27, 19–34 (first part, 19–27).

Murray, C. & Frenk J. 2000. A framework for assessing the performance of health systems. *Bulletin of the World Health Organization*, 78, 717–731.

Chapter 8

Technology and Health

Learning Objectives

- Define health technologies and discuss their relevance for health and health systems.
- Describe the stages of technological innovation: how a health technology is invented, selected, initially adopted, produced, goes into widespread use and is adapted or retired.
- Discuss the benefits of health technologies and how they can be expanded.
- Discuss the potential harms of health technologies and how they can be mitigated.

8.1 Introduction

Advances in information and communications technology (ICT) have been called the Fourth Industrial Revolution, with the potential to transform work, family and social bonds, education, politics and certainly health. From diagnosing cancer through artificial intelligence (AI) to robots providing home care for the elderly, from digitizing health records to chatbots answering health questions online, there is a wide range of ways in which technology is shaping health and will continue to do so. This is not just a recent development. Rather, technology has enabled advances in public health since the inception of the field.

In this chapter, we take some time to delve into the concept of technology and its relationship to health. We first propose a definition of health technology, drawing upon previous definitions of technology but also health actions and health systems. We then examine why technology matters for health, by analyzing one of the most famous public health debates in recent years: what role did medical technologies such as vaccines or antibiotics play in the spectacular twentieth century's epidemiological and demographic transitions that we discussed in Chapter 6?

Next, we describe the stages of the innovation process, drawing upon previous models by Anadon et al. (2014) as a way to understand how health technologies are invented, selected, initially adopted, produced, go into widespread use and are eventually either adapted or retired.

We conclude this chapter with a discussion on the benefits and potential harms of health technologies, looking more particularly at the rise of AI and its applications in health systems in recent years.

8.2 Defining Health Technologies

Harvey Brooks defined technology broadly as "knowledge of how to fulfil certain human purposes in a specifiable and reproducible way" (Brooks, 1980). Technologies can profoundly affect health – positively or negatively – whether or not health is their intended purpose. Consider, for example, how the internet facilitates access both to beneficial health education and to harmful disinformation. Consistent with our definition of a health action (see Chapter 7), we can understand health technologies as a subset of technologies where the **primary intent** of their use is to improve or maintain health. We can then paraphrase Brooks to conceptualize health technologies as knowledge of how to protect or promote health in a specifiable and reproducible way. The World Health Organization (WHO) has similarly recognized knowledge as core to the concept of health technology, which it defines as "the application of organized knowledge and skills in the form of medicines, medical devices, vaccines, procedures and systems developed to solve a health problem and improve quality of life" (World Health Organization, n.d.). Defined in this way, knowledge that contaminated water spread cholera in London in 1854, and that disabling the water pump handle could slow the outbreak – known as the birth of epidemiology – can be seen as an early public health technology (Tulchinsky, 2018).

It may be intuitive to think of health technologies as tangible goods, such as medicines or hearing aids, in which case the knowledge is embodied in a physical product. But as the definitions above suggest, knowledge of how to protect, promote or restore health in a specifiable and reproducible way can also focus on less tangible outputs, such as procedures and systems. For example, monitoring the growth of a child according to a standardized growth chart is a specifiable, reproducible way of tracking their health and development, alerting caregivers when something is amiss. Health technologies can be both tangible and intangible, or a combination of both.

The availability of health technologies can transform how we understand health. Consider the discovery that a class of diabetes medicines (i.e., glucagon-like peptide-1 [GLP-1] agonists such as semaglutide, known by its trade names Ozempic and Wegovy) help people who use them lose weight. For better or worse, obesity has to some extent been reframed from what some considered an issue of personal responsibility into a health condition amenable to medical intervention (Warin et al., 2024).

Access to health technologies, such as vaccines against deadly diseases like measles, can also mean the difference between life and death, between good or poor health. Where access is equitable, health technologies can alleviate the health effects of poverty and reduce inequalities. Conversely, when access to an essential health technology is delayed or denied, it can deepen divides between the haves and the have-nots (see examples later in this chapter). Thus, health technologies raise important ethical, social and political questions, which we explore further below.

8.3 The Role of Technology in Health Improvement

As we saw when we discussed the epidemiological transition (Chapter 6), since the twentieth century there has been an unprecedented improvement in health conditions around the world. The most dramatic summary of such improvement lies in the fact that life expectancy has more than doubled during this period. It is only natural, then, that many researchers and scholars have devoted their work to accounting for the main drivers of such a major transformation. In particular, there has been a vigorous debate about the relative weight of health technologies versus broader determinants of health.

Although it has a long history in medicine and public health, this debate was intensified by the interest in accounting for the impressive mortality reductions achieved during the last century. Such reductions have benefited practically all countries of the world and all social groups, although with enormous disparities in the extent and pace of progress. The coincidence in time of this process with the multiplication of efficacious medical technologies led to the almost obvious conclusion that the latter had to be the cause of the reduction in mortality. Yet this certainty was not to last long (Frenk, 1998).

In the decade of the 1950s, precisely at the time when most countries were beginning to report important decreases in mortality, several influential criticisms were leveled against the conventional wisdom. In 1959, René Dubos published his now-classical book *Mirage of Health* (Dubos, 1959). There, he demonstrated that mortality had begun to decline in the West before the formulation of the microbial theory of disease and the availability of "magic bullets." Almost at the same time, the physician and demographer Thomas McKeown was beginning the series of studies that would make him one of the most controversial critics of the role of medicine (McKeown, 1980). According to McKeown, the main reasons for the decline of mortality were to be found in better living conditions, especially nutrition, housing and environmental sanitation. This was certainly not the first time that the effect of social conditions on health had been noted (an observation that goes back at least to the Greeks and that finds an eloquent exponent in Rudolf Virchow). The important point, however, was that both Dubos and McKeown were specifically trying to refute the common notion that medical technologies were responsible for major gains in health.

Medical intervention has always been accompanied by skepticism about its value. But what began to be expressed in this debate were not doubts about particular interventions but about the entire health care enterprise, leading to what Paul Starr has called a new "therapeutic nihilism." This view implied a radical shift in public policy for health. Whereas a common policy goal throughout the world had been to achieve universal access to health care, the notion of the relative irrelevance of care undermined the rationale for such a goal. As Starr points out, if medical services make so little difference in health and life expectancy, ". . . why worry about the poor – or, for that matter, anyone – not getting enough of them?" (Starr, 1976). The irony is that therapeutic nihilism began as a critique from the left but was subsequently incorporated into the conservative justification for cutting health care budgets and tolerating socioeconomic inequalities in access.

Today, we recognize that the debate between medical technologies versus socio-economic development as alternative determinants of health improvement represents a false dilemma. Health services and their associated technologies are not disconnected from social conditions, as the debate often seems to suggest. On the contrary, the quality and coverage of health services are an integral part of the definition of development itself and constitute one of the main indicators of social well-being. Sustained health improvement would appear to be the result of a process of development that includes access to high-quality services as one of its main components.

A major step forward toward this integrative perspective was the work of demographer Samuel Preston, whose research led to what has come to be known as the "Preston curve" (Preston, 1975). This depicts the relationship between life expectancy and income per capita for different countries. Not surprisingly, as income per capita increases, so does life expectancy, although this is a curvilinear relationship with diminishing returns

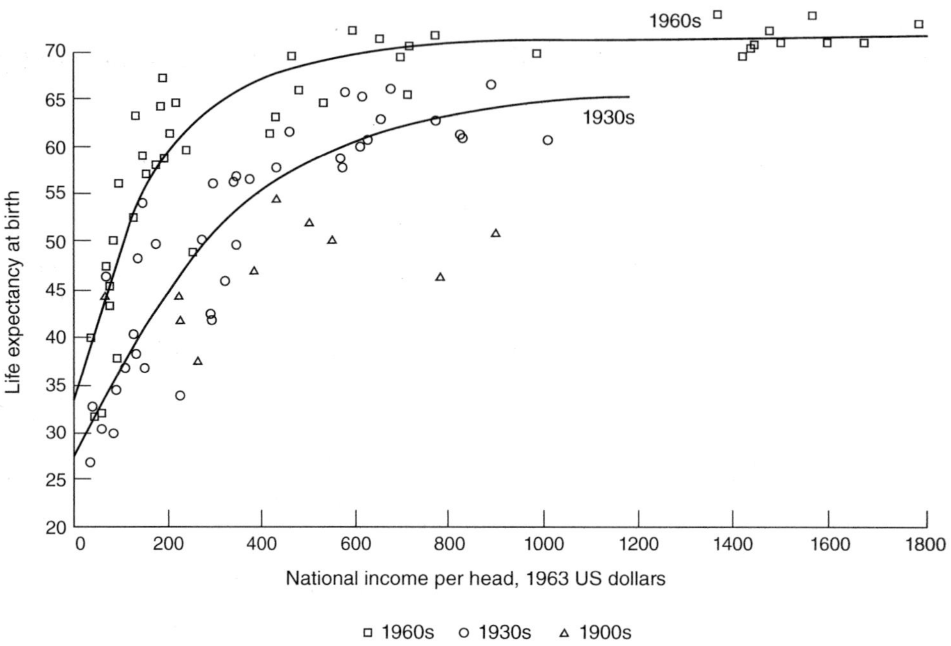

Figure 8.1 Preston curve of the 1900s, 1930s and 1960s.

as countries get wealthier. Preston's crucial insight arose when he plotted the curve for successive decades of the twentieth century and found that there was an upward shift in the curves. This means that the same level of inflation-adjusted income per capita (on the x-axis) yields increasingly higher levels of life expectancy (on the y-axis) at each successive decade. His model, copied in Figure 8.1, displays a scatter plot illustrating the relationship between these elements in the 1900s, 1930s and 1960s. The gap between the lines plotted along 1930s and 1960s data points holds space that accounts for the increase in knowledge around the globe, consequentially contributing to increased life expectancies and improved economic conditions.

In Figure 8.2, we present a Preston curve modeling the cross sections of adjusted net national income per capita in current US dollars and life expectancy at birth in 1990 and 2020 using World Bank data.

If we think of income per capita as a summary measure of economic development and life expectancy as a summary indicator of health in a country, Preston's finding provides an integrative solution to the false dilemma mentioned earlier. The positive relationship between life expectancy and income per capita reflects the effect of social conditions on health improvement. At the same time, the upward shift in the curve reveals that a substantial proportion of health improvement is not explained by growth in real income per capita, since in each successive decade the same income produces a higher life expectancy than in the previous decades. That difference represents the influence of exogenous factors, primarily the role of knowledge (as opposed to general socioeconomic development) on health improvement.

There are three main mechanisms through which knowledge improves health. First, as we saw earlier, knowledge gets translated into new technologies, such as vaccines,

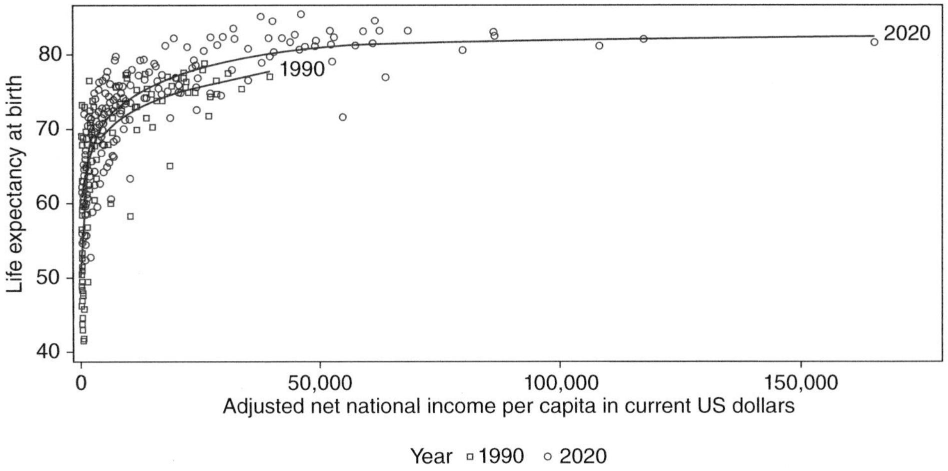

Figure 8.2 Preston curve of 1990 and 2020.

drugs and devices. This is the best-known mechanism through which it improves health. Second, knowledge is also internalized by individuals, who use it to structure their everyday behavior in key domains like personal hygiene, feeding habits, sexuality and child-rearing practices. Finally, knowledge becomes translated into evidence that provides a scientific foundation both for health care and for policy formulation. This explanation acknowledges the central importance of health technologies in health improvements, while also stressing the centrality of advances in education that empower persons to be co-producers of their own health and the key role of evidence-based practice and policies. Based on the work by Preston and subsequent authors, it is estimated that more than half of the gains in life expectancy since the twentieth century have been due to advances in knowledge.

The lesson is clear: we must supersede false dilemmas if we wish to understand and act upon the intricate causal web that determines the improvement of health conditions and their distribution across social groups. Health is too complex a process to allow one-sided conceptions and prescriptions. Removal of structural social barriers that limit opportunity, promotion of healthy behaviors and universal access to high-quality services powered by technological advances are not alternative but synergistic strategies in the pursuit of better health.

8.4 The Importance of Technology for Health Systems

In Chapter 7 on complex systems, we identified technologies as one type of resource that health systems need in order to function (alongside human resources, payment mechanisms and scientific information). In this framework, technology development can be understood as a critical resource generation activity.

Technology plays a crucial and often contradictory role in health systems. First, while technologies have always had an important place in public health, they are arguably playing an increasingly salient role in daily life in nearly all parts of the world. They hold tremendous potential for transforming and improving health systems. For example, digitizing a patient's health records so that a team of physicians and nurses understands their history can improve the quality and continuity of care. Patients can save considerable time, money and get access to specialized experts through telemedicine. As Blumenthal and Kong highlighted during the COVID-19 pandemic, technologies were critical for combating the virus – from vaccines to masks, from contact tracing to physical distancing (Blumenthal and Kong, 2021). Therefore, these authors argued that the capacity to develop and effectively deploy technologies ought to be considered a new kind of essential public health infrastructure. Second, the globalization of trade and travel, and the speed at which information and ideas move across borders, have intensified the opportunities and challenges that technologies raise for public health. For example, knowledge of how to protect health that is developed in one place, such as a medicine to cure hepatitis C, can be transported and made available in another – a powerful conduit for expanding the benefits of new knowledge for public health. On the other hand, knowledge that comes with risks or even causes harm can also spread widely through a technology, such as disinformation on the safety of vaccines or the marketing of infant formula as a replacement for routine breastfeeding.

Finally, there is a complex mix of actors involved in the development of technologies ("resource generation" as we referred to it earlier), including universities and other research institutes, public and private research funders and private firms. More than in many other parts of the health system, the role of private firms is particularly pronounced in technology development, production, marketing, sales, adaptation and retirement (Røttingen et al., 2013). To make matters more complex, technology can enhance the effectiveness and efficiency of health care, but it can also lead to duplication, waste or outright misuse. This reality has prompted the creation of specialized agencies in most countries to assess benefits and weigh risks and harms to govern how firms are permitted to sell many health technologies in the market. The role of private firms and arrangements for public stewardship of the market are a hallmark of health technologies that are critical to a fuller understanding of public health.

Below, we provide a conceptual framework for thinking clearly about how technologies are developed and deployed. We also pose two key questions to structure how we may think about their role in public health: How can the benefits of health technologies be expanded? How can their risks and harms be appropriately governed?

8.5 Stages of Technological Innovation

How do new technologies get developed and eventually impact individual or population health? Or, returning to the definition of technology above, how does knowledge come to be "specified" and "reproduced"? Brooks defined technological innovation as "the process by which technology is conceived, developed, codified, and deployed" (Brooks, 1980). It can be useful to conceive of the innovation process as comprised of stocks and flows, occurring across seven stages, as illustrated in Figure 8.3. (The figure and remainder of this section draw heavily from Anadon et al. (2014).)

We begin on the left side of the figure with a stock of **knowledge** that can grow continuously through contributions from basic research, traditional and experiential knowledge. As noted in the Preface, knowledge is continuously produced and reproduced and can be utilized to invent new technologies (stage 1). Invention can be the result of goal-oriented research, such as when a firm seeks to develop an improved diagnostic test for COVID-19. Or it can result from accidental discovery, such as when a

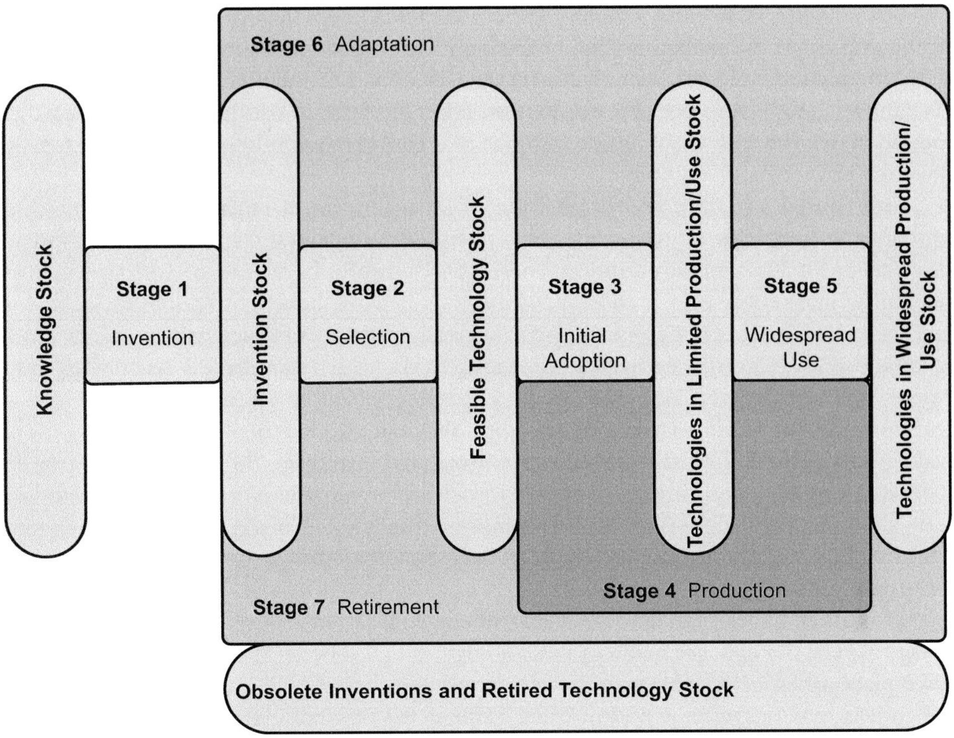

Figure 8.3 Seven stages of technological innovation.

desirable and/or profitable side effect is discovered during pharmaceutical testing, as occurred when researchers using botulinum toxin to treat an eye disorder observed that it could also smooth facial wrinkles, a potentially lucrative aesthetic application (Monheit and Pickett, 2017). Inventions can also be the result of repurposing a pre-existing technology; for example, when an antibiotic drug developed to treat one type of bacterial infection is demonstrated to be effective against another.

Once inventions enter the **invention stock**, a selection process takes place in which some, but not all, inventions are chosen for further advancement (stage 2). Selection can be done directly by potential users, such as when a consumer selects and downloads a newly invented application for use on their smartphone. It can also occur through policies such as regulatory standards or national objectives (e.g., declaring malaria elimination to be a national goal), which permit or promote some inventions over others. Finally, selection is also often done by agents who select on behalf of principals – that is, users. For example, a regulatory agency can be seen as an agent that applies standards to select which health technologies are considered safe and effective enough to be made available to potential users in society. Similarly, a health care provider, such as a physician, nurse or pharmacist, can be seen as an agent who selects which medicines are appropriate for a patient, the principal.

After a technology is selected it enters the **feasible technology stock** from which technologies are initially adopted and/or produced. Initial adoption (stage 3) can be the result of many factors, such as marketing, the spread of information about an invention, the benefits offered to early adopters or a price that is lower than pre-existing competing technologies. At the same time, the invention must be produced or reproduced (stage 4). For tangible technologies, manufacturing is necessary. For intangible technologies, such as handwashing before surgery, **production** takes the form of codification, such as a sign posted above the sink in all health facilities of a country reminding users of the steps to take for proper handwashing.

After initial adoption and production of an invention, it enters the stock of **technologies in limited production/use**. From here, some inventions move into widespread use (stage 5). Like initial adoption, there can be multiple drivers of widespread use, including marketing, information, advantageous pricing, benefits to adopters, behavior and culture. Of note are network effects, "when a product or service gains value as more people use it" (Oxford Learner's Dictionary, 2024), which can drive a technology into wider use in a society. An example of a network effect is when more people use a communication platform (e.g., WhatsApp, WeChat, X, Facebook), it becomes more valuable to others to use the same platform and increases the costs of leaving it, perpetuating adoption of that platform into widespread use. Notably, widespread use can also be impeded by lack of information, disadvantageous pricing, behavior and culture, limiting the extent to which society benefits from a health technology (see Section 8.6.1 for further discussion).

Two other stages span across several others: adaptation and retirement. **Adaptation** (stage 6) refers to changes made to a technology so that it better meets needs, and it could take place when a technology is invented, selected, initially adopted, produced and/or when it is in widespread use. Non-users, such as the original inventor or another party, may adapt the technology, such as when a company issues a new version of its computer software that has improved features over the previous version. End-users themselves may also redesign a technology, or learn how to make better use of it, such as when programmers adapt open-source software to better meet their specific needs. Technologies may also be **retired** (stage 7). This can take place relatively early, for example, when an invention is not selected, perhaps because it was considered too risky or there was no profitable market for it. Retirement can also take place after a technology is initially adopted or enters widespread use. Drivers of retirement include risk assessment, decreased demand, unfavorable pricing, poor performance or harm revealed once a technology is adopted at scale. For example, some medicines that appeared relatively safe during clinical trials on a few hundred patients are revealed to have unacceptably harmful side effects once they are used by thousands and/or for longer periods of time, and regulators may require they be withdrawn (retired) from the market.

These seven stages can be applied to a wide range of technologies – including but not limited to health technologies – and this conceptual framework is intended to facilitate clear thinking about how a technology may or may not progress through these stages to impact health.

8.6 Challenges for Technologies and Public Health: Expanding Benefits and Mitigating Risks and Harm

Societies must grapple with two interrelated challenges when it comes to technologies: how to expand their benefits and mitigate risks and harm. Many technologies are neither purely beneficial nor purely harmful for health, but rather, a mix of both. For example, chemotherapy can drive cancer into remission but cause serious side effects for patients undergoing it. A smartphone app can track the user's physical activity and motivate a more active lifestyle but also increase exposure to privacy breaches or advertisements with misleading health information. An enduring challenge is how to expand the benefits of technology so that more people can benefit from advances in science and health-related knowledge and, at the same time, manage the risks that technologies may pose and mitigate harm. We address each of these in turn.

8.6.1 Expanding Benefits

The "right to enjoy the benefits of scientific progress and its applications" was included in the 1948 Universal Declaration of Human Rights and the 1966 International Covenant on Economic, Social and Cultural Rights, but has until recently been a relatively neglected topic in the human rights field (United Nations Committee on Economic, Social and Cultural Rights, 2020). Growing attention to this right reflects, arguably, the increasing salience of technology to multiple dimensions of human life as well as the rising profile of political debates on who should or does benefit from technological advances. There is a strong moral argument that expanding the benefits of *health* technologies, in particular, deserves special attention because they can profoundly shape the life chances and capabilities of individuals, including determining whether they enjoy better or worse health, whether they live or die.

The centrality of knowledge to health technologies has two important implications: that it is *eminently possible* to expand access to its benefits through more open sharing of knowledge but, at the same time, the need to find ways to pay for knowledge creation and development often places *limits* on its use.

Knowledge can be a global public good if it is made openly, publicly available. That is, in theory, everyone can benefit from new health-related knowledge (it is non-excludable) and one person consuming that knowledge does not reduce the amount remaining for others to consume (it is non-rival), meeting the two essential characteristics of public goods (see also discussion of public goods in Chapters 7 and 12). Returning to our earlier examples, the use of growth charts to track a child's health over time or handwashing protocols in health care facilities are both technologies whose benefits are publicly available to anyone who would like to make use of them. Other intangible technologies, for example, code for health-education software, could also be a public good if it is made openly available, as is the case with open-source software. Tangible technologies such as medicines can be understood as comprised of both a physical component (e.g., a tablet) and a knowledge component (e.g., the demonstrated knowledge that 300 mg of a particular chemical ingested once per day safely and effectively treats a particular infection) (Moon et al., 2017). The cost to develop a new medicine is essentially the cost of generating this kind of knowledge, and can be understood as distinct from the costs to manufacture the tangible product.

Indeed, inventing or adapting new technologies entails costs, which may be borne by different actors including a university, government, private firm or individual. Inventors may seek to put a price on that technology to recover those costs or earn a profit. The central rationale of patents and other intellectual property rights is to incentivize invention by enabling inventors to recover the costs and potentially profit from sales of their invention during time-limited state-granted monopolies (Mazzoleni and Nelson, 1998). Patents have become a central legal institution that structures and provides economic incentives for the development of many pharmaceuticals (they are present but play a less central role in other areas of health technology such as medical devices or software). However, patents and other monopolies can also restrict production, enable the seller to charge high and/or unaffordable prices, and constrain follow-on innovation. Because of the important distributional implications, some of the longest running and heated debates in global health concern the appropriate level of patent protection in different situations (e.g., such as pandemics) or for countries at different levels of economic development (World Trade Organization, 2020).

Expanding the benefits of health technologies poses the societal challenge of selecting which technologies to provide, to whom, and how to manage the costs of doing so. Unequal access to the benefits of health technologies, both within and across countries, can exacerbate inequalities and, where avoidable, are inequitable. Lack of access to HIV treatment in most low-income and middle-income countries at the turn of the millennium sparked a global political movement that successfully mobilized international funding and flexibility in intellectual property rules ('t Hoen et al., 2011), cutting deaths from HIV by 69% from their 2004 peak of 2.1 million, to 630,000 deaths in 2022 (World Health Organization, 2023). As technology advances and offers the possibility to address previously intractable health conditions, persistent and difficult questions remain regarding who will benefit from them. For example, gene therapy that can prevent progressive blindness comes with a high price tag (Takagi, 2023) – $342,000 per dose per eye in Japan in 2023 – raising concerns about access, affordability and the sustainability of health systems (Morgan et al., 2020).

Specialized agencies mandated to conduct a "comprehensive evaluation of the consequences of a medical technology" (Fineberg, 1985) – health technology assessment (HTA) bodies – have been established in many countries over the past several decades to provide systematic analysis that informs technology selection and pricing or reimbursement; examples include the United Kingdom's National Institute for Health and Care Excellence or Thailand's Health Intervention and Technology Assessment Program (Tantivess et al., 2017). HTA bodies may consider many aspects of a technology, including technical performance, safety and efficacy, cost, efficiency, acceptability to patients, research value and ethics together with broader effects on the health care system, on households and society (Fineberg, 1985). Such assessments can inform a wide range of decision-making, such as whether a technology should be adopted by the health system, who should benefit from the technology (especially if rationing is required) and what prices the system should be willing to pay. Other tools, such as formularies or national lists of essential medicines, reflect the need to select and prioritize public spending among a growing list of potential technologies.

Health technologies raise a range of complex and difficult ethical questions. For example, when health technologies are scarce, who should get priority and on what basis? Or when a technology offers both significant benefits and great risks, as with novel experimental products, how can genuine informed consent of users be ensured? Guidance from ethics committees can help decision-makers in such situations. For example, when global demand for a new malaria vaccine exceeded supply, the WHO issued guidance in 2022 on how to allocate the vaccines ethically both across and within countries, taking into account principles such as greatest need and expected health impact (World Health Organization, 2022d). The ethical issues raised by health technologies touch on some of the most fundamental questions facing societies, regarding autonomy, respect, fairness, justice and solidarity.

8.6.2 Mitigating Risks and Harm

On the other side of the coin from benefits lie the risks and potential harm of technologies. Health harm can be caused by a wide range of technologies, such as accidents caused by driverless cars or plastics pollution from industrial manufacturing processes. Not all technologies are subject to regulation, and approaches to regulation vary widely by country.

Health technologies – though intended to protect, improve or restore health – can also cause harm, such as substandard poorly manufactured medicines or emerging large language models reinforcing existing racial or sexist bias. The highly consequential, complex nature of health technologies means they are usually scrutinized and regulated more tightly than other technologies. Most countries have specialized regulatory agencies to continuously assess the safety, efficacy and quality of health technologies. Examples include the US Food and Drug Administration at national level and European Medicines Agency or African Medicines Agency at regional level; approval from such regulators is often required before a health technology may be sold or used in a country

Since the turn of the millennium, in limited cases the WHO has also gradually taken on functions similar to those of regulatory agencies, to support more resource-constrained agencies and/or to make assessment more efficient. For example, the WHO Pre-Qualification Program assesses the quality of manufacturing of priority products such as vaccines and drugs for reproductive health, HIV, tuberculosis and malaria; a dossier assessment or site visit to a manufacturer conducted by the WHO can be far more efficient than dozens of national regulators doing the same. The WHO also makes recommendations on whether candidate products should be used during emergencies through its emergency use listing procedure; it can be much faster for the WHO to assess and provide a public opinion on a dossier submitted by a product developer, as occurred with COVID-19 vaccines during the crisis, than for each national government to assess applications filed by a range of developers (Ravinetto et al., 2024).

The WHO does not replace national regulators, who are ultimately responsible for decisions to permit use of a health technology in their territories and must often make context-specific and value-based judgments on whether a technology's benefits outweigh the risks of harm. It is this context specificity that is also a point of debate, as some argue that international regulatory harmonization is needed to accelerate assessment processes and lower the cost to product developers of obtaining regulatory approval in a wide range of countries. However, others argue that a unified regulatory standard cannot meet the needs of countries with vastly different disease burdens, health systems, values and cultures – and, therefore, different risk–benefit trade-offs. The consequences of regulatory standards can be significant, especially if they act as barriers to entry for new competitors (Berman, 2017).

A perennial challenge facing regulators, and governments more broadly, is how best to regulate novel, emerging and/or disruptive technologies, such as AI or human genome editing. Policy-makers face a well-documented range of challenges: information asymmetry in which the product developer has far more information than the regulator;

Box 8.1 The rise of artificial intelligence: a challenge for health systems

The wide-ranging health implications of AI illustrate well the challenges of regulating emerging technologies. AI chatbots can provide health information that may be helpful or misleading. AI companions may alleviate loneliness or harm the mental health of adolescents. AI-driven analysis of large datasets can accelerate drug discovery. AI-empowered facial recognition software may also perpetuate biases, or provide more accurate results for some racial groups versus others. AI may improve the efficiency of health care workers by replacing the need to perform repetitive tasks or reduce important human interactions with patients. Beyond the health sector itself, AI could have transformative and disruptive effects on many of the social determinants of health, such as education, employment, transportation and political processes.

Societies face major challenges in regulating AI. AI developers usually have a much better understanding of the potential and risks of their technologies, creating a situation of information asymmetry for regulators. There is considerable uncertainty about both the potential benefits and harms of AI across many uses and population groups, such as children or older adults versus more tech-savvy young adults. And there seem to be no simple solutions for how to regulate this dynamic and complex technology, such that regulation has lagged behind AI, illustrating well the "pacing problem." Some governments hesitate to regulate AI companies or applications, considering AI an important sector for economic growth and military advantage vis-à-vis competitors (Taeihagh, 2021; Bode et al., 2023).

In light of these difficulties, analysts have called for "governing" AI rather than "regulating" it, with regulation seen as a subset of the broader concept of governance. The Organisation for Economic Co-operation and Development (OECD) defines governance of technologies as "the process of exercising political, economic and administrative authority in the development, diffusion and operation of technology in societies," involving not only governments but also firms, civil society and communities of practice. Governance of AI could take place throughout the life cycle of the innovation process (i.e., invention, selection, production, initial and widespread adoption, adaptation and retirement), and simultaneously across multiple levels – local, national and international. Governing AI is seen as more effective than traditional regulation for steering the direction of this technology, though many questions remain on how exactly to do so (Gill, 2021).

the "pacing problem" in which regulation nearly always lags technological development, and uncertainty about both the risks and harm technologies may cause as well as the efficacy of solutions proposed to address them.

This set of challenges requires a difficult balance between committing type I errors – over-regulating technologies and thereby denying people their benefits – or type II errors, under-regulating technologies and exposing people unreasonably to risks and harm. Traditional regulatory approaches (e.g., risk assessment, product-based standards, liability) can be too little and/or too late for the scale of impacts of emerging technologies (Taeihagh et al., 2021; OECD, 2024). In addition, existing health regulators, having traditionally focused on drugs and diagnostics, might not be well equipped to assess emerging health technologies such as AI or blockchain technologies (see Box 8.1). There is an active, ongoing debate on what mix of traditional and novel approaches to governing technologies may be most appropriate in this Fourth Industrial Revolution (Gill, 2021).

8.7 Summary

Health technologies are essentially knowledge of how to protect or promote health in a specifiable and reproducible way. Most of the dramatic improvements in life expectancy during the past century have been fueled by better knowledge, which gets translated into specific technologies, while also empowering persons to be co-producers of their own health and illuminating practitioners and policy-makers with scientifically derived evidence. Technologies are becoming increasingly salient tools for protecting and promoting public health but can also come with significant risks or cause harm. Technological innovation is not just the process of inventing a new technology, but rather, should be understood as the process by which a technology is invented, selected, initially adopted, produced, goes into widespread use and is adapted or retired. Expanding the benefits of health technologies is feasible because of their core knowledge component. Doing so can be a moral imperative, especially when they can alleviate suffering and save lives. But costs, information, culture and other barriers can prevent the benefits of health technology from being widely available. HTA bodies can inform decision-making on how to expand the benefits of such technologies. Societies must also find ways of mitigating the risks and harm that health technologies can pose, and they have traditionally relied on specialized regulatory agencies to assess whether a technology's benefits outweigh the risks in order for it to be authorized for use. The rapid pace of technological innovation raises challenges for traditional regulation, however, prompting the need for new approaches and perhaps for policy experimentation in how best to ensure and expand access to the benefits health technologies may provide while protecting society from their potential harm.

Comprehension and Discussion Questions

- Give an example of a tangible health technology and an intangible health technology. What should be considered a technology – that is, what are the boundaries of the concept?
- At which stage of the technological innovation framework would you position recent innovations such as telemedicine, AI-powered health apps or malaria vaccines?
- What criteria do you think governments should consider when selecting which technologies to invest in developing? To purchase?
- Choose a technology that has implications for health. In your country or state/province, how adequate is regulation of this technology to ensure fair access to its benefits? To address its risks or harms? What more could be done to improve regulation or, more broadly, how it is governed?

Chapter 9

Health System Performance

Learning Objectives

- Analyze the concept of health system performance.
- Discuss different ways to assess such performance and their potential benefits and drawbacks.
- Relate overall performance with the performance of subcomponents or organizations in health systems.
- Distinguish between vertical and horizontal integration of health systems and relate these variations to overall system performance.
- Discuss how factors external to health systems affect performance, and consider how to deal with them.
- Analyze the role that leadership, institutions, systems design and technologies play in health system improvement.
- Examine how to assess the performance of intermediate levels, taking into account productivity, quality and accessibility.

9.1 Introduction

In Chapter 7, we posed five key questions on the fundamental elements that define a health system. There, we addressed the first three questions dealing with boundaries and actors, goals and functions. We now address the remaining two questions by examining the relationships among those fundamental elements, in an effort to understand the performance and characterize the specific organizations that comprise the health system.

Most of this chapter is based on work done at the World Health Organization (WHO) to undertake the first comprehensive assessment of health system performance in all countries. The results were published in the 2000 edition of the WHO's flagship publication, the *World Health Report*, which that year was titled *Health Systems: Improving Performance* (World Health Organization, 2000). To date, this report remains one of the most cited publications by the WHO. It generated an extensive set of rankings, which operationalized elements of the conceptual framework (referred to at the beginning of Chapter 7) that was developed by Christopher Murray and Julio Frenk, both working at the WHO then. The exercise was, by its very nature, controversial. Some countries which ranked low in the comparative indicators responded in a defensive manner, but many others (such as China and Mexico) used evidence of relatively poor performance as motivation to carry out deep reforms that generated important improvements. This outcome provides reassurance that rigorous conceptual formulations often lead to practical applications with positive impact on the health and well-being of millions of persons. It also underscores the need to compare the performance of different health systems facing the same challenge in order to learn lessons from the best performers that may prove valuable to the rest. Chapter 14 presents such a comparative performance analysis regarding the widely differing responses by Japan and the United States to the COVID-19 pandemic.

9.2 How Good Is a Health System's Performance?

We now turn our attention to the fourth question in our framework: how good is a health system in terms of its performance? While performance is an essential concept when discussing health systems, it is not as simple as simply recording the level of goal attainment. We need to define the scope and boundaries of such performance, as well as the standards to which we compare it.

9.2.1 Goal Performance, Composite Goal Performance and Efficiency

With a clearly defined set of goals and their measures, we can compare the level of goal attainment for different health systems. There is a long history of comparing measures of health across countries. The concept of performance, however, is more complex than simply recording the level of goal attainment. Performance of the health system involves relating goal attainment to what can be achieved. In other words, performance is a relative concept. A high-income country has higher levels of health than a low-income one, but which country has a higher level of performance relative to health system resources? We argue that performance should be assessed relative to the worst and best that can be achieved for a given set of circumstances.

Figure 9.1 illustrates the concept of performance with respect to the goal of improving population health. The y-axis shows health, and the x-axis shows resources spent on the health system. The top line shows for populations A and B the maximum attainable level of health for each level of health expenditure, given the non-health system determinants such as the level of education. It is clear from the figure that performance is related to the level of health expenditure; for example, population A has a lower level of health than B, but the two populations have approximately the same level of performance.

Measuring goal performance is intricately related to the question: Does one hold the health system accountable for the level of key determinants of health that are not entirely

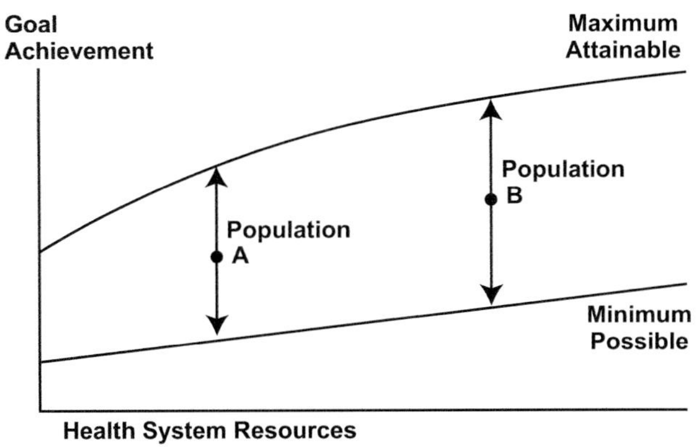

Figure 9.1 The concept of performance. Reproduced from *Bulletin of the World Health Organization*, Vol. 78, No. 6, Murray, C. J. & Frenk, J., "A framework for assessing the performance of health systems," pages 717–731. Copyright (2000).

the responsibility of the health system but can be influenced by it? We argue that the answer must be yes. The health system should be held accountable for these broader determinants of health to the extent that the best health system can influence them as compared to the worst health system. Some might argue that we should not judge the performance of health systems to be poor simply because the population level of tobacco consumption is high, leading to low levels of health. The implication of this argument is that health systems should not be held accountable for the levels of determinants such as tobacco consumption, diet or physical activity. Yet the counterargument is strong: a good health system should pay attention to the level of tobacco consumption or the composition of the population's diet. In operationalizing the concept of performance, careful attention should be paid to the determinants or the fraction of determinants that the health system should be routinely held accountable for and those it should not. For example, health systems should be held substantially accountable for the levels of tobacco consumption; the health system should probably be held much less accountable for levels of educational attainment.

The criterion that should be used to determine the extent to which the health system should be held accountable for a determinant of health is the degree to which the best health system can change the level of that determinant. This degree is related to the time frame of the analysis. What the health system can achieve in one year to reduce tobacco consumption is different from what the health system can do in five or ten years. Should assessments of performance be made compared to what the best health system could do in one year compared to the starting point at the beginning of the year? We argue that performance assessment should be undertaken with a longer time horizon. The maximum level of goal attainment achievable at a given level of health expenditure should include what can be achieved over many years. Otherwise, health systems are never held accountable for past mistakes nor rewarded for past successes. As one of the purposes of performance assessment is to provide a firmer empirical basis for the analysis of key organizational factors influencing performance, performance measurement should not be overly sensitive to the starting point for a given year. Many health sector reforms and institutional changes may take several years to achieve their full effect, requiring a longer-term perspective for assessment.

Performance can be assessed for each of the health system goals described in Chapter 7, that is, the level and distribution of health improvement and health system responsiveness as well as financial fairness. In other words, by choice, a society may perform poorly on responsiveness but well on health inequality because more resources from the total budget are assigned to addressing health inequalities than to enhancing responsiveness. Ultimately, a single budget for the health system is used to achieve all the goals. Because there will be implicit or explicit trade-offs between some of the goals, performance in achieving the composite of the three goals is also a useful construct. In economics, the concept of efficiency means producing a desired output at least cost, or producing the maximum quantity for a fixed budget (Boadway and Bruce, 1984). More formally, production efficiency is based on the concept of a Pareto optimality in which factors of production are allocated in such a way that it is not possible to reallocate factors so as to produce more of one good without producing less of another. In this sense, composite goal performance – how well a health system achieves the desired outcomes given available resources – is also the efficiency of the health system. We will use interchangeably the term composite goal performance and efficiency in the rest of this chapter.

As noted in Section 7.4 on health system goals, societies may value the five components of the three goals differently. The function relating attainment on each goal to overall goal attainment represents an important policy choice that each society must make for itself. Nevertheless, we believe that there will not be great variance in the importance attached to different goals for most societies in the world. Shared conceptions about the importance of these goals will allow for meaningful comparisons between countries of the performance on each of the five components of the three goals and on composite goal performance (Bok, 1995). These comparisons will provide an empirical basis for debates on the effect of different patterns of health system organization. By facilitating these comparisons of performance and efficiency, the framework proposed here can enrich the policy debates on the design, organization and operation of health systems.

Measuring performance and efficiency using a common framework does not mean that one particular health system design will emerge from the analysis as a blueprint for all countries. Nevertheless, it can help assess how policy choices and organizational design can affect health system outcomes, as illustrated by the case of Costa Rica, given in Box 9.1.

Box 9.1 Costa Rica: story of an outlier

A small middle-income country in Central America, Costa Rica is often presented as a public health exemplar thanks to its outstanding health outcomes. In 2022, its life expectancy at birth was almost the same as its Northern neighbor, the United States, at 77.3 years versus 77.4 years, despite a gross national income per capita five times less (World Bank Group, 2022a). Its infant mortality rate, an indicator often considered to be a tracer for health system performance, is 6.5 deaths per life births, half the one for Latin America and the Caribbean (13.5 in 2022) (World Bank Group, 2022b). Most striking is the speed of its decrease: in 1965, this same indicator was estimated to be at 70 deaths per live births: a 10-fold decrease in just 60 years.

Part of this success can be attributed to economic improvement: the country has benefited from stable economic growth, democratic stability and little inflation for the most part of the twentieth century and is widely considered a development success story. But this explanation alone would be too simplistic (Unger et al., 2008). In fact, studies have found that up to 75% of the reduction observed in infant mortality could be attributed to Costa Rica's health services (Rosero-Bixby, 1991).

An analysis of this success points primarily to the creation of a unified social security system, the Caja Costarricense de Seguridad Social (CCSS), in 1941 and the deployment of a highly successful primary health care model, strengthened in the 1990s through a series of reforms. Costa Rica has established a comprehensive network of multidisciplinary teams, deployed in all regions, focused on providing disease prevention, community health education and home care as well as first-level clinical care (Pesec et al., 2017).

Not surprisingly, Costa Rica was able to deploy a rapid, coordinated response to the COVID-19 pandemic thanks to its integrated approach to health care delivery, and its established infectious disease control program (Prado et al., 2024).

In summary, Costa Rica illustrates well the concept that performance of health systems is relative to a country's level of income and/or health expenditure. Wide variations can be observed even at similar levels of economic development, as in the comparison of Costa Rica with the Latin American region, and health attainment can be similar at very different levels of resources, as in the comparison between Costa Rica and the United States.

9.2.2 Performance of Subsystems or Organizations

The performance of the entire health system must be related to the performance of various subcomponents or even organizations such as hospitals or institutions offering population health services within the health system. Work on the performance of providers of personal health services is converging with work on overall performance assessment of health systems. Our conceptual framework for performance presented for the entire health system is largely applicable to subcomponents such as the public health services or to specific organizations such as a hospital or outpatient care provider. The key would be to compare the level of goal attainment for the entire population to the level of goal attainment that would be achieved with the best and worst performance of that subsystem or organization. Of course, the operational challenge will be how to define the best and worst attainable lines for a given subsystem or organization.

This mapping from the framework for the overall system to its subcomponents will work well for the level of health and responsiveness. The potential contribution of any one organization to the distributional goals will be much smaller and much more difficult to estimate. As this health system performance assessment framework is developed and implemented, further work on its application to organizations and subsystems will need to be elaborated.

It is also important to note that the applicability of the approach to specific organizations or subsystems does not imply that the overall performance of the system is a simple (additive or even multiplicative) function of the performance of different subsystems or organizations. Interactions between, for example, the performance on intersectoral activities to reduce exposure to tobacco through excise taxes and the performance of hospitals and clinics will be highly complicated. It may ultimately not be possible or even useful to try to define the relationship between overall performance and the performance of various subsystems or organizations.

9.3 How Do We Relate Architecture to Performance?

Now that we have examined the concept of performance, we turn our attention to the relationship between health system architecture and performance. More specifically, how we relate architecture to performance. Understanding this relationship obviously matters when designing and reforming complex health systems.

9.3.1 Vertical Integration

As indicated earlier, health system performance is related not just to the organization of each separate function but also to the way in which each function relates to each other. For example, vertical integration whereby one entity is responsible for more than one function is the norm, not the exception. The extent of vertical integration may matter for some combinations such as revenue collection and purchasing or purchasing and provision, but not for others. Figure 9.2 illustrates four different polar examples of vertical and horizontal integration or segmentation of financing, provision and stewardship functions. In this figure, each box represents an organization that undertakes one or more functions. The horizontal axis represents coverage of the population.

In the vertical and horizontal integration model, the functions of financing, provision and much of stewardship are integrated into a single public sector organization covering the entire population. The United Kingdom National Health Service before the reforms

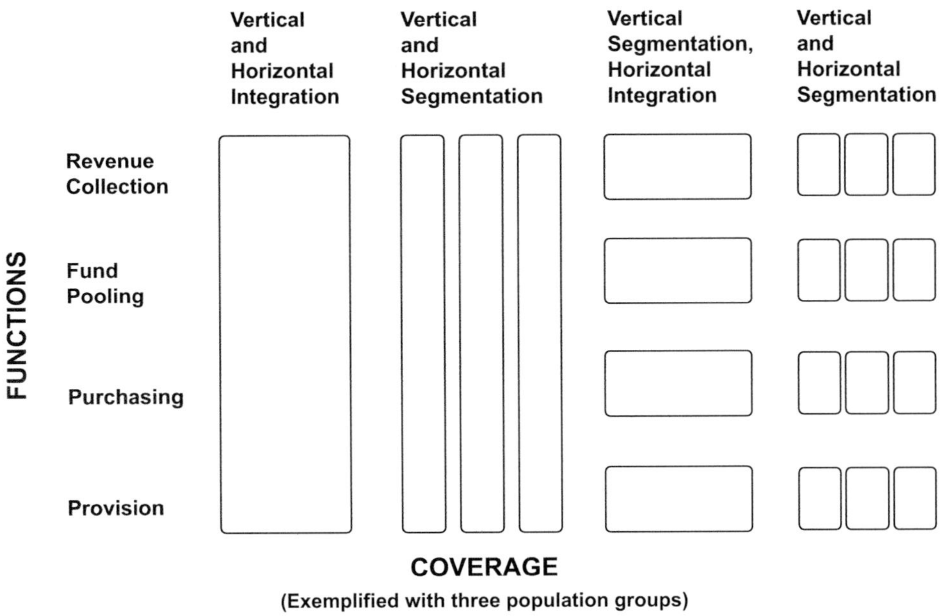

Figure 9.2 Health system models, according to types of integration. Reproduced from *Bulletin of the World Health Organization*, Vol. 78, No. 6, Murray, C. J. & Frenk, J., "A framework for assessing the performance of health systems," pages 717–731. Copyright (2000).

of Margaret Thatcher was somewhat close to this degree of complete integration. Figure 9.2 also illustrates a system with vertical integration but horizontal segmentation; different organizations, each integrating the financing and provision functions, cater to different population subgroups. Examples that approximate this model include the segmented systems of much of Latin America. Figure 9.2 also illustrates two other models. One is vertical segmentation and horizontal integration, examples of this degree of functional specialization by organizations including Australia, Colombia and several autonomous communities of Spain. In fact, many of the current reform proposals aim at this type of functional organization of the health system. The most atomized health systems, where there is vertical and horizontal segmentation, are also illustrated.

A key policy question is the extent to which functional specialization or integration affect health system performance.

9.3.2 Factors External to the Health System

The discussion so far of factors influencing health system performance has focused on the organization of five basic functions of health systems – financing, provision, stewardship, systemic integration and resource development – and the extent to which they are vertically integrated. There are, however, factors outside of the health system that will influence the performance of these functions. These are aspects of the organization of other social systems. For example, the presence of an effective judicial system may have a substantial influence on the ability of purchasers to enforce contracts on providers. General attributes of government, such as ethical codes of conduct and the tolerance of corruption, may influence the performance of stewardship and other functions as well.

These interrelationships stress that some ultimate determinants of health system performance lie outside the formal architecture of the health system.

One main concern for those who work on health system performance is the scope of accountability for health systems. Simply put, should a health system be accountable narrowly for actions within its organizations or more broadly for key determinants of goal attainment outside the boundaries of the health system? Two viewpoints can be articulated: (i) it is unfair to hold health systems accountable for things that are not completely under their control; and (ii) health systems can achieve greatest impact through influencing non-health system determinants of health. Through our framework for health system performance assessment, we confront this debate in three ways.

First, by describing the levels of health system goal attainment, regardless of the reasons that explain them, national and world attention can be brought to bear on which countries have done well in improving health, reducing health inequalities, enhancing the level and distribution of responsiveness and financing the system in a fair manner.

Second, as discussed earlier, the assessment of relative performance should include how well a country is doing on controlling the level of non-health system determinants to the extent that a good health system can influence the level of these determinants through effective intersectoral action. The ultimate reason why we must include to a lesser or greater extent these non-health system determinants is that if the health system is not held accountable for them, no one will be the advocate in a country for addressing these issues. The best hope for change in many cases lies with the health system's ability to articulate the importance of addressing these problems. Problems such as tobacco consumption, diet and unsafe sexual activity must be included in the assessment of health system performance. The potential for the health system to influence other determinants such as educational attainment, general social inequalities or biodiversity is much less, and the assessment of health system performance should reflect this fact.

Third, for the assessment of the performance of specific subsystems and individual organizations, the scope of accountability is much narrower. Broad accountability for the non-health system determinants of health belongs with the overall health system. Performance assessment for components of the system naturally narrows the scope of accountability to those actions directly influenced by the subsystem or organization in question.

By approaching the problem at these three levels, we feel that we can focus attention on overall attainment of health system goals, the performance of national health systems and the performance of specific subsystems and individual institutions.

By clearly distinguishing the intrinsic goals of health systems from the organization of different functions of the health system and the technical content of the provision of personal, hybrid and public health services, we hope to facilitate a more constructive dialog on health policy. There has long been a debate over whether health system architecture matters more or less than the intervention mix delivered by the systems. Interventions must be delivered by health systems and health systems without effective interventions are useless. These two worldviews should not be seen as competitive but rather as complementary. By introducing clear measurement of health system goal attainment and performance, key aspects of the organization of health system functions and the technical content of health service provision, we hope to facilitate a more reasoned and informed debate on the interaction of system architecture and intervention mix.

Much of the debate on health system design is couched in claims and counterclaims about what works and what does not work. The only support for some claims may be theoretical models or anecdotal evidence. Many economists defend health policies with basic utility models; for example, if consumers are perfectly informed and providers are competitive, then user fees will enhance efficiency (World Bank, 1987). Other analysts often defend their claims with anecdotal evidence of one or two health systems. Given the extraordinary diversity of health system organization, for every anecdote there is often a counter-anecdote. Few decision-makers or health system experts have access to information on many different systems and their levels of achievement.

Implementing the ideas developed in this and previous chapters for health system performance assessment will lay the basis for a shift from ideological discourse on health policy to a more empirical one. Over time, we should be able to provide empirical answers to such questions as the relationship between the organization of health financing and the level and distribution of health and responsiveness. This line of work should make it possible to ascertain the extent to which, for example, competition among purchasers or providers enhances responsiveness. If the framework encompasses the main intrinsic goals for health systems and the key candidate factors for explaining variation in performance, it will lay the basis for a more scientific discourse on health policy.

Annual assessments of health system performance will focus attention on the policy options available to governments for improvement. Global institutionalization of performance assessment may contribute to the ongoing reflection on the role of the State in health systems. What policies can enhance performance? What evidence is there that the State can enhance performance through the adoption of these policies? An enlightened role for the State then becomes to enhance performance where the evidence supports its potential to do so.

This framework for health system performance assessment is work in progress that will undoubtedly evolve as its operationalization proceeds and evidence accumulates on the link between health system structure and performance. The development of such a long-term agenda will help countries all over the world articulate a better response to the complex and changing health needs of their populations.

9.4 A LIST for Health Systems Improvement

We know that there are wide variations in performance by different health systems, even at the same level of income per capita and health expenditure. These variations are due to the influence of several determinants enclosed in the acronym **LIST**, which stands for **leadership**, **institutions**, **systems design** and **technologies**. These determinants are enumerated in decreasing order of complexity, from the bottom up.

9.4.1 Technologies

No health system can succeed if it does not deliver the appropriate set of interventions, along with their accompanying technologies. This is the aspect that has been better studied and where we have substantial consensus on priorities. Most development cooperation for health has been directed to expanding the supply of drugs, vaccines, bed-nets and other technologies. However, to work at all, these technologies must be embedded in the second element.

9.4.2 Systems Design

Quality services can only be delivered if a set of subsystems (such as procurement, information, personnel, etc.) are designed so that the required structures and procedures can assure the timely conjunction of human, financial, technological and knowledge resources. One positive aspect of the global initiatives on health system strengthening is that they address many of these crucial issues. But it is also necessary to take the next step in our acronym.

9.4.3 Institutions

Development is only possible through the patient construction of institutions, which represent the vehicles whereby human beings mobilize their talents, values and interests toward the pursuit of shared goals. Institutions also introduce certainty to transactions and articulate incentives. In addition to hospitals, clinics, educational centers and research organizations, a crucial institution is the ministry of health. Despite its central importance for the stewardship function, many countries are far from having an optimal ministry of health. In this regard, there seems to be a sharp contrast with ministries of finance, where the imperatives of globalization have imposed a fairly homogeneous level of technical proficiency across countries. Ministries of health should certainly be sensitive to local realities, but there is a technical core that is increasingly connected to global networks and should therefore be strengthened through global efforts. Proficient stewardship is essential to achieve good performance in the face of the pluralism that characterizes most health systems in the world, whereby a diverse set of public and private providers of services coexist. If it is to yield positive results, such a mixed participation requires clear stewardship that can set fair rules of the game and a level playing field for all actors. Whether it involves ministries, hospitals or academic centers, institution building is always tough because it requires long-term investments that are often obliterated by short-term political pressures. This problem is related to the last element in the LIST.

9.4.4 Leadership

Probably the most complex challenge in health systems is to nurture persons who can develop the strategic vision, technical knowledge, political skills and ethical orientation to lead the complex processes of policy formulation and implementation. Without leaders, even the best-designed systems will fail. We come back to this point in Chapter 13.

9.5 The Role of Global Institutions

The present moment offers a unique opportunity to advance specific proposals on each of the four elements of health system strengthening: greater access to life-saving technologies, improvements in critical subsystems, long-term investments in institution building and leadership development. So far, global organizations have paid attention mostly to the development of technologies – an effort that clearly must continue. As stated earlier, at least part of the global interest in national health systems has centered around challenges related to personnel, logistical and information subsystems. This is a move in the right direction, but it should be expanded to include a concerted effort to strengthen ministries of health, build other crucial national institutions and deploy a wide-ranging program for identifying, training, nurturing and supporting present and future leaders.

For these investments to be successful, they must be linked to concrete health outcomes. In this respect, global health requires a new way of thinking and acting in order to bridge the traditional divide between the "vertical" approach, focusing on technical interventions for specific disease priorities (Garrett, 2007), and the "horizontal" approach, aimed at strengthening the overall structure and functions of the health system but without a clear sense of priorities. The solution is a truly "diagonal" approach, whereby explicit intervention priorities are used to drive improvements into the health system (Sepúlveda, 2006).

A major obstacle to effective global action, as we will argue in Chapter 12, is the weak coordination that characterizes the institutional architecture for global health. There is a contradiction in the fact that the current interest in national health systems has not been accompanied by a parallel interest to develop a true global health system. The very international institutions that purport to assist countries to develop integrated and coherent national health systems have themselves been incapable of adopting such attributes for the inchoate global health system that today is characterized by inefficient duplication of certain functions, neglect of others and imposition of high transactions costs on countries where multiple programs operate. Yet, when it comes to health systems, there is a dialectic of mutual support between the national and the global levels. The global health system can only achieve results through well-performing national health systems, which themselves require a functional and harmonized global system that can be truly supportive of national development.

9.6 Performance at the Intermediate Level: Programs and Organizations

Up until now, we have been discussing health system performance at the macro level, looking at the entire architecture of health systems. Now, we are going to spend some time focusing on an intermediate level, at the specific programs and organizations where these goals and functions get carried out and active services are delivered.

Our point of departure is a modification of the model developed by Avedis Donabedian, which we saw in Chapter 3, when we discussed health needs. The first step in the organized social response is when society takes a subset of health conditions and decides that the subset requires care and therefore becomes a health need. Once health needs are defined, services must be produced to meet those needs, and resources must be deployed. One of Donabedian's fundamental insights is that the relationship among health needs, services and resources is not direct but mediated (Donabedian, 1973).

We are going to look at what happens after that initial step.

Figure 9.3, a modified version of a diagram by Donabedian, shows us with the dashed arrows that when we're planning services, we first must diagnose the needs; then plan what services would meet those needs; and then plan for the resources we'll need to produce those services. In the evaluation stage, shown by the dotted arrows, we go the other way around, evaluating how productive resources were in generating services. Most of the time the analysis stops here but, ideally, it is necessary to take the last step and evaluate how well the provided services meet the original needs.

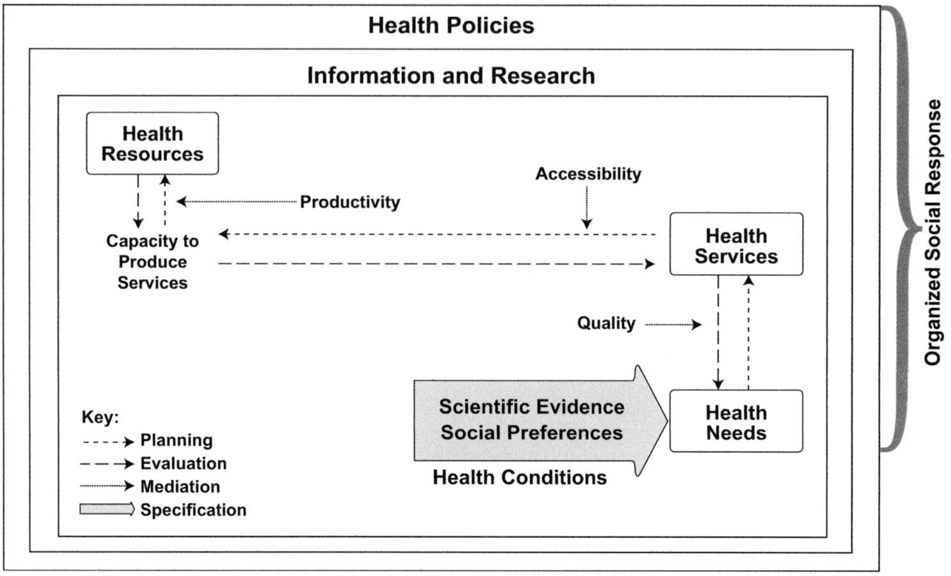

Figure 9.3 Substantive areas of public health.

As we see in Figure 9.3, there are three mediating resources: productivity, accessibility and quality. Productivity is defined as the relationship between inputs and outputs expressed in physical units. Some examples include the number of patients per physician or nurse; the number of hospital discharges (an output) per hospital bed (a resource); the number of surgical procedures (an output) per operating theater (a resource).

Productivity is not enough, however. It determines a potential capacity to produce services, but we cannot stockpile services. By definition, the moment of production and moment of consumption occur at the same time in "services," as opposed to "goods," where they are not simultaneous. When it comes to health services, there may be the capacity to provide services, but if those resources are not accessible to the population, then production doesn't happen, and services are not provided.

The most important health resource is people, but can also include equipment, medications and so forth. When it comes to human resources, we can study what factors determine productivity, such as age, gender and level of training.

Accessibility illustrates very nicely the idea that the health system is best understood as the relationship between the population and a set of institutions including providers. Accessibility is an attribute of the degree of fit between the characteristics of the resources and the characteristics of the potential users of the services. Is the clinic available? Are there doctors and nurses in the clinic? Is the equipment there and functioning? Availability is necessary but not sufficient, because available resources must also be accessible. If the fit is off, utilization doesn't happen, and the services cannot be considered accessible.

Geographic accessibility is the first and most obvious type of accessibility: where is the clinic or service located relative to where the people live? Accessibility here is a measure of the fit between the spatial distribution of resources and the spatial distribution of the population.

Financial accessibility is another key factor. If we say the services are unaffordable, we are saying that they are not a good fit given the distribution of wealth (of resources) in the population.

Cultural accessibility is also very important. If you have a clinic where the providers only speak English located in a community where people speak other languages, there's no fit. Beliefs can also play a role. If the local population thinks that diseases are caused by forces of nature and providers have a more Western scientific view, there is a lack of fit. Public health officials can preach and prescribe all they want, but there will likely be a high likelihood of low adherence with medical services with this misfit, or the services may be utilized, but they will not be aligned with what is important to the population.

The fourth form is **organizational accessibility**. One of its key dimensions refers to time distribution. If the opening hours of a clinic do not match the distribution of free time, such as clinics that are open exactly when children are at school and grownups are at work, or when you have long waiting times during open hours, you have a bad organizational fit. The distribution of time on the resource side as well as the population side determines organizational accessibility.

There is also what we might call **psychological accessibility**. This could include the physical safety of a clinic not being in a war zone or a dangerous neighborhood. It could also relate to stigma. You might not want to be seen going to an AIDS clinic or an addiction rehabilitation center. The extent to which a facility creates a safe environment both from physical dangers as well as stigmatizing threats is a very important dimension and a good example of this notion of degree of fit.

Finally, one last form is **statutory accessibility**, that is, the lawful exclusion of particular groups from receiving care. Statutory accessibility refers to the institutional framework of legal or political elements that impact the availability of health care to individuals. This concept defines various restrictions or limitations to provisions of accessible care through legislation written by governing bodies. This could include, for example, restricting access to safe abortions, reproductive health care, gender-affirming care or harm reduction services, as well as restrictions targeted to specific categories of the population, for example, undocumented migrants, or in specific geographical areas.

Once a resource is available and it fits the corresponding characteristics of the population, then utilization happens. Most of our evaluation stops there – we delivered so many babies, etc. But that is not enough. In public health, we need to take the last step related to the very important notion of quality of care. Meeting the need is a function of the quality of service. Quality is better understood, as Donabedian explained, as having a technical and interpersonal dimension. We tend to focus on the technical dimension, which itself has two fundamental aspects: the safety and the effectiveness of services. Safety means the services do not produce harm. The worst level of quality is when it produces harm (Jha et al., 2013) due to negligence, lack of skill, organizational factors, etc. When quality is negative, instead of addressing a need, utilizing services leads to new needs. The level of quality here refers to the optimal balance between the risk and benefit of a service. When quality is good, the benefits override the risks and care is effective, producing the result we want, which is an improvement in health. A big challenge to the measurement of quality is trying to ensure that it can be attributed to care. Quality has been defined as the difference between what's achievable with current technology and what's actually achieved with the services we deliver (Donabedian, 1973). If a patient has an incurable disease from which he or she dies, that is not an example of a lack of quality, because a cure was not currently achievable. Quality lies between the frontier of possibilities defined by the level of technology (what is achievable) and what we actually achieve.

But quality is not just technical; it has, as discussed in Chapter 7, an interpersonal dimension too. Responsiveness to the legitimate expectations of the population is an intrinsic goal of the health system, and the extent to which it is met reflects the interpersonal dimension of quality. This dimension includes both respect for the rights of patients associated with their care and what we called in Chapter 7 the consumer orientation of services. When quality is high, we both meet the patient's needs through effective treatment, and the patient is satisfied. Satisfaction is a subjective state, which is a product of system responsiveness. In turn, high interpersonal quality feeds back into technical quality, with patients more likely to adhere to therapeutic interventions if they feel they are well cared for.

What Donabedian calls the medical care process (see Chapter 3) does not happen in a vacuum. Health personnel provide information, including about the availability of services, and research offers an understanding of cost-effectiveness and capacity. This all happens in a framework of policies. The process is not fixed, but instead it is time and space dependent. There are policies and regulations about all the elements and relationships shown in Figure 9.3: needs, services, resources, and the mediating factors that make it possible to plan and evaluate health care.

It is hard to think of any other industry that offers as many services as the health system. These services range from true public goods to what economists call private goods. In public goods, one person's use of the good doesn't take away from another person using it, such as epidemiological surveillance. If we have good surveillance, it benefits everyone. An example of a strictly private good would be the removal of your appendix. It is only yours. There is also a range around repetitiveness of use. You acquire information about products by consuming them repeatedly. Then there are services where patients lack information from prior consumption. Hopefully, a patient who comes into a hospital suffering from a heart attack has never had one before, and that patient wants to be treated in a way so that they will never have one again. There are also predictable treatments, such as elective surgery, and emergencies where there is no predictability. Such heterogeneity of services is one of the key challenges for health system performance.

9.7 Summary

In this chapter, we have focused on two questions regarding health systems. The first question concerns how good a health system is in terms of its performance. Performance of the health system involves relating goal attainment to what could be achieved in a given set of circumstances and is therefore a relative concept. There are wide variations in performance by different health systems, even at the same level of income per capita and health expenditure. Health systems can be strengthened through attention to four elements (LIST): leadership, institutions, systems design and technolgies.

The second question concerns how we can relate health system architecture to performance. The architecture of health systems varies widely across countries. A health system can be integrated or divided across segments of the population, or by function (e.g., revenue collection, pooling, purchasing, service provision and stewardship). Relating architecture to performance is a central question for the study of health systems. Health systems assess needs, and then mobilize resources to provide services. How well the system performs in doing so depends on three mediating factors: productivity, accessibility and quality. Productivity is defined as a relationship between inputs and outputs expressed in physical units. Accessibility can include geographic, financial, cultural, organizational, psychological or statutory factors, and is necessary for a population to utilize services. Finally, the quality of services matters – that is, the difference between what's achievable and what's actually achieved with the services we deliver.

Next, we turn our attention to a sixth question: How do health systems change?

Comprehension and Discussion Questions

- What is the concept of relative performance described in this chapter? How is it different from absolute performance? Provide an example (real or invented) to illustrate your point.
- How does the overall system performance relate to the performance of subsystems or organizations?
- In this chapter, we propose four elements (simplified as the LIST) to strengthen health systems: leadership, institutions, systems design and technologies. Do you think those elements are sufficient? Why or why not?
- Should a health system be accountable for non-health system determinants of health? Why or why not?

Papers from Which This Chapter Is Adapted

Frenk, J. 2010. The global health system: strengthening national health systems as the next step for global progress. *PLoS Medicine*, 7, 1–2.

Murray, C. J. L. & Frenk, J. 2000. A framework for assessing the performance of health systems. *Bulletin of the World Health Organization*, 78, 717–731.

Chapter 10

Health System Dynamics

Learning Objectives

- Identify different types of health systems, and how they vary by the degree of State involvement, the functions performed by governments and which population groups are eligible to receive services.
- Identify and provide examples of different types of power that operate in policy processes.
- Explain processes by which health policies may undergo significant change, using two well-known policy frameworks: Kingdon's multiple streams framework and Sabatier's advocacy coalition framework.

10.1 Introduction

Just as health conditions change, as we saw when we discussed the demographic and epidemiologic transitions, health systems also transition. Health systems are complex, their change over time will also be complex, and there is still much we do not fully understand. This chapter provides frameworks for thinking about the drivers and ways in which health systems change.

The first step in understanding the dynamics of health systems is to develop a classification for the main types of health systems, so we can then understand how they evolve. If you look today at the landscape, we see very different types of health systems around the world. The classification developed here relies on a relational framework, which you may remember as the relationships among the main actors, including citizens, providers and the government.

The second step is to explore the way through which policies undergo changes. For this, we explore two aspects of policy changes. (i) We look at the different types of power in health systems, and the way through which actors leverage their power to enact change. (ii) We analyze the way policies change, drawing upon two well-known theories in political science: Kingdon's multiple streams framework and Sabatier's advocacy coalition framework.

10.2 Modalities of State Involvement

It should be clear from the formulation in Figure 7.2 that the State is not a unidimensional or homogeneous actor. Apart from its strictly regulatory and mediating role, the State may act as a health care provider (when it is involved in the direct delivery of services) or as a source of financing (e.g., when it runs social insurance funds).

Furthermore, there are many public agencies that are not part of the health system per se, but that constitute a key element of its institutional environment. This is the case of the legislative and judicial branches of government, as well as the executive offices dealing with public budgets, taxation and law enforcement. We may conclude, therefore, that the State occupies multiple positions in the health system and its environment.

The precise configuration of State involvement is a key feature to differentiate various types of health systems. Many typologies attempt to classify the entire health care system by taking the country as the unit of analysis. This is often not possible, because the State may participate in more than one way within a given national system. Although useful for broad comparative purposes, aggregate classifications encompass, under a single category, total health systems that have, in many cases, a mixture of different forms of State intervention. For example, the British National Health Service is a composite of two quite different modalities: one for general practice, where the State finances the care that is provided by private contractors, and another for specialty care in hospitals, where governmental organizations directly provide services.

It is better to use a lower level of aggregation than the whole country to classify health systems (Frenk and Donabedian, 1987). We call this lower level a "modality," by which we mean a particular configuration of State involvement in regulation, financing and delivery of health services related to a specific principle for population eligibility.

Based on our model of the components and relationships of health systems, as explained in Chapter 7, it is possible to derive a typology of health system modalities. This typology is presented in Table 10.1. Unlike earlier attempts, which have tended to focus solely on the supply of services, the proposed classification follows a relational perspective derived from our definition of a health system, which includes the population in its structured relationships with a set of institutions. Thus, each modality results from combining a level of State control with a population eligibility principle.

Like any classification, this one represents an abstraction from real-life complexities. As a result, it concentrates solely on the central axis of health systems, namely, the relationship between the providers, the population and the State. This does not imply that the remaining actors identified in Chapter 7 – the resource generators and the other

Table 10.1 Typology of health system modalities

Functions performed by the State (degree of control)	Basis for population eligibility			
	Purchasing power	**Poverty**	**Socially perceived priority**	**Citizenship**
Stewardship	Private enterprise	Private charity	Company-based services	Social insurance (German model)
Financing		Medicaid (United States)	Incipient health insurance	National health insurance
Delivery		Public assistance	Social security (Latin American model)	Socialized (national health service)

sectors that influence health – are not important, but that their different forms of organization are compatible with several types of modalities and are therefore not essential to the classification.

A clarification should be made regarding the names of the modalities shown in the cells of Table 10.1. In order to ensure a degree of continuity with earlier literature on the subject, conventional terms, such as "national health insurance" or "national health service," have been preserved. However, earlier uses of these terms were applied to total health systems; in contrast, they are used here to designate a modality that may coexist alongside others within a health system.

Apart from making it possible to identify the modalities that are present in a given country, the typology can reveal certain international patterns. It can be seen, for example, that not all modalities are equally probable. Thus, the State does not usually finance or provide services when eligibility is based solely on purchasing power. (Through subsidies and tax deductions, the State can indirectly finance private care, but these situations do not represent health system modalities.)

Another very infrequent modality restricts the role of the State to financing health services for people with lower incomes. One of the very few contemporary examples is the Medicaid program in the United States. The lack of other cases could reflect the fact that, in trying to subsidize the assimilation of people with lower incomes into the private care system, such modality goes against the common practice of providing health services for people with lower incomes through a separate, State-owned modality, such as public assistance.

Apart from those modalities that have been adopted only infrequently or not at all, there are others that are now rare but were common in the past. Such is the case of company-based services, under which private employers organize the financing and delivery of services for their workers (Soberon et al., 1986). As compulsory social insurance expanded, this modality was largely displaced, although it has not yet disappeared completely; for example, it is still found in the United States.

The typology also has the advantage of differentiating situations that are usually grouped together in more conventional classifications of total health systems. The most important case refers to the different social security modalities shown in Table 10.1. In their incipient stages, many social security schemes were directed exclusively at workers earning less than a specified wage. Their dependents were usually excluded, as were the self-employed, the peasantry and the middle and upper classes (Institute of Medicine (US) Committee on Employment-Based Health Benefits, 1993). This modality can still be found today in certain Asian and African nations that have recently introduced national health insurance reforms (Lagomarsino et al., 2012). In the case of Europe, coverage was progressively extended to broader groups, until the citizenship principle was adopted. Even so, there are still differences regarding the degree of control. In Germany, for example, financing is handled by private, non-profit funds that contract private providers. The State is restricted to regulating these two groups and to establishing the minimum levels of benefits to which all citizens are entitled. In almost all other Western European countries, service delivery remains in private hands while the State has taken charge of finance, thereby giving rise to the modality generally known as national health insurance. Two important exceptions are Great Britain and Sweden, where the State has been directly responsible for the delivery of most services; therefore, the dominant modality is socialized care, also known as a national health service (Starr, 1982). As indicated previously, in almost all these countries there have also been other modalities.

10.3 Segmented Model

One prime difference between countries is, precisely, the degree of fragmentation of State involvement in health as measured by the number and relative strength of modalities (Murray and Frenk, 2000). In this respect, it is necessary to distinguish two forms of fragmentation. In the first one, the various coexisting modalities may deal with different types of services, but each of them covers the entire population, as in the British case. In the second one, modalities are fragmented by population subgroups, as in many Latin American countries, where the government owns and operates two distinct subsystems: on the one hand, public assistance for the rural and urban poor, who are self-employed, unemployed or altogether out of the labor force; on the other, social security, mostly for wage earners. This sort of segmentation usually has negative effects on equity, since the modalities that take care of people with lower incomes end up having fewer resources to cope with a larger burden of health needs. Given the polarized character of the epidemiological transition, such arrangements reproduce social inequality. That is what has happened in most Latin American countries with a bimodal public sector, to which one must add private providers that concentrate resources on the care of the better-off groups. Rather than being pluralistic, these are polarized systems.

In the twentieth century, most health systems in Latin America (and some in other developing regions) were organized by population groups. This "segmented" health system model segregates the various social groups in different institutional niches (see Figure 10.1).

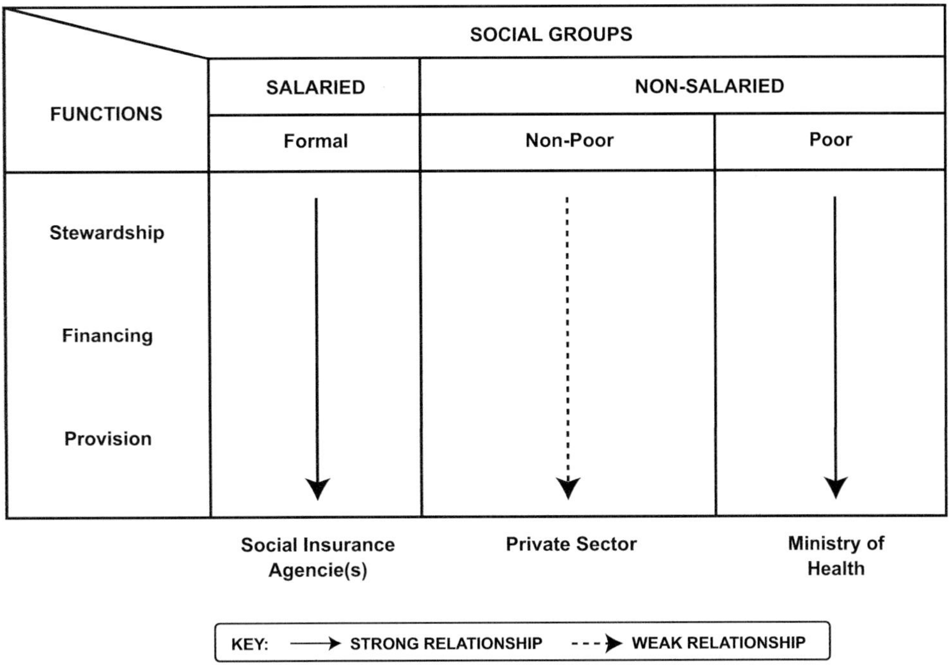

Figure 10.1 Health system design by segmentation of social groups.

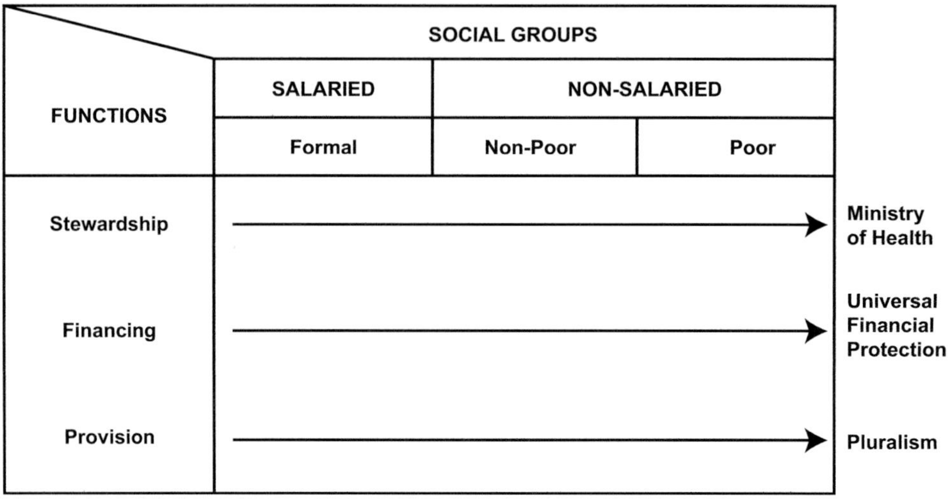

Figure 10.2 Health system design by separation of functions

The ministry of health provides health services to the non-salaried poor; social insurance agencies to the salaried workers of the formal economy; and the private sector to those with the capacity to pay. Each institutional segment performs the stewardship, financial and provision functions, but focused only on a segment of the population. In sum, this model is characterized by vertical integration of functions with horizontal segregation of population groups.

This way of organizing the health system has proven to be inequitable, inefficient and unresponsive. It provides unequal benefits, levels of quality and degrees of financial protection to the different social groups, even within the public sector. It generates undesirable duplicities and resource waste. Given the monopoly power of each institution in the provision of services, it also tends to be indifferent to the needs and expectations of service users.

In recent decades, several countries in Latin America (and other developing regions) have been moving away from the segmented model by organizing their health systems by functions, rather than population groups (see Figure 10.2). In this new scenario, the three essential health system functions (stewardship, financing and delivery) are performed for the population as a whole. In counterpoint to conventional segmentation, this emerging model is characterized by horizontal integration of population groups with separation of functions. The stewardship function is performed by the ministry of health, which assumes responsibility for strategic planning of the system as a whole and guarantees a balanced relationship among all actors through the design of adequate rules and incentives. The financing function is performed by one or a few public funds, which should eventually provide financial protection to all the population. Finally, the delivery function is performed by a plurality of providers, public and private, under the supervision of a regulatory body (Frenk, 2015).

In an earlier article (Londoño and Frenk, 1997), we called this emerging model "structured pluralism" with the intention of underscoring the need to find a middle ground between the polarized health system arrangements that had been implemented throughout Latin America. With the word "pluralism" we looked to avoid the extremes both of public monopolies and the atomization of the private sector, while the word "structured" underscored the need for strong State participation, not as a monopolistic provider but, as mentioned above, as a steward responsible for providing strategic direction, assuring fair financing and enforcing transparent rules of the game. Health systems in the region have been moving at a very different pace in this direction, and even those countries that more explicitly adopted this model (Colombia, Chile and Mexico) need to further strengthen the integration of population groups and the separation of functions. They also need to resist recent policy attempts to return to earlier forms of segmentation. We will come back to this topic when we discuss health system reform in Chapter 11.

10.4 Hypothetical Pathways

With some additional refinements, our typology can also be used to search for regularities in the historical development of health systems. One approach to studying the historical experiences of different groups of nations is to perceive the relationship of the State to the providers of care, on the one hand, and to the populations, on the other, as a dynamic process. To do so, these two dimensions must be conceptualized as continuous variables that characterize a country as a whole. The total impact of State intervention (including all its modalities) can be represented by the proportion of the population covered by all public programs. Similarly, the degree to which a State controls the means for producing health services can be represented by the proportion of all personal health care expenditure (both public and private) that is incurred through modalities characterized by State ownership.

Assuming the necessary information is available, it should be possible, by treating the extent of State control and population coverage as continual, to plot, for a particular country, the historical changes in these two features of State intervention in health care. Countries could then be grouped according to similarities in their historical developments. Of course, each country will have its own peculiar path. For example, most Western industrialized countries have first increased their population coverage, with the State relying heavily on the private sector both for the delivery of services and for the administration of benefits through existing sick funds. Here, the extensions of more direct State control, beyond the functions of financing and enforcing the compulsory enrollment of successive population groups in an insurance plan, largely came about only after a high percentage of the population was already covered. The example of Taiwan given in Box 10.1 illustrates this pathway.

On the other hand, generally speaking, low- and middle-income countries have done things in a reverse way. With a few exceptions, State intervention in these countries was not based on the use of private resources; these remained in a separate system for providing medical care to those who could afford it. Instead, the State created its own network of facilities and providers to take care of relatively small segments of the population that had access to the public system because they had lower incomes, had contributed to a fund or were made the privileged beneficiaries of State action. Only after

Box 10.1 State interventions: an example of recent reform

Taiwan introduced its National Health Insurance (NHI) in 1995, which provides universal mandatory coverage to its citizens and permanent residents. The NHI replaces a system which previously included more than 10 public insurance schemes for specific population groups, and which only covered 59% of the total population. Delivery is contracted out, mostly to private providers. Stewardship for the overall system is done by the Ministry of Health and Welfare, which oversees the NHI administration. Private health insurance policies exist only for disease-specific cash indemnity provisions, for example, for private hospital rooms or devices not covered by the NHI. In this example, a large portion of the population was already covered by health insurance prior to 1995, but the State increased its coverage by making enrollment compulsory (Tikkanen et al., 2020). This is an example of a country moving toward a national health insurance system, organized by functions rather than by social groups, where the government concentrates on the financing and stewardship functions, while contracting out health care delivery.

a State-owned system was in place did these countries start extending the provision of services to a larger part of the population.

Even though they are based on a fair number of observations, the proposed paths of State intervention should be considered as only hypothetical. One would need a more thorough empirical investigation to determine whether these paths truly reflect the historical experiences of State intervention and, if that is the case, to specify not only their precise trajectories, but also the rates at which countries have moved along them.

10.5 Theories of Policy Change

In addition to understanding the characteristics of various types of health systems as they evolve, it is also important to understand the political processes by which health systems change. Why did the Affordable Care Act become law in 2010 after decades of unsuccessful efforts to expand insurance coverage in the United States, and what shaped its contents? What forces made it possible to achieve universal health coverage in Mexico by 2012, as discussed in Chapter 11? How did Thailand's pioneering anti-smoking policies get put in place in the late 1980s (Vateesatokit, 2003)? Who shaped the amendment of India's patent law in 2005 to make medicines more affordable (Kapczynski, 2009)? To begin unpacking these questions, it may be instructive to review concepts of political power, actors and theories of policy change.

Processes of health system change can involve hundreds of actors, including various parts of government (legislatures, courts and executives at federal, State and local levels), private firms, academic experts, civil society organizations, such as patient or advocacy groups, and the media, among others. Each of these actors will have deeply held values and interests that may compete or conflict with each other. Policy processes can play out over long or multiple time periods, sometimes spanning decades. They may take place at various levels of government (or governance, when there is an absence of clear governmental authority as at the international level), sometimes simultaneously. Finally, more than many other areas of policy, health policy tends to involve highly complex issues, such that technical knowledge and actors with technical expertise are often quite influential. To start making sense of this complexity, it can be useful to simplify the system by examining its components, beginning with power and actors.

10.6 Power and Actors

To understand these policy processes, it is useful to consider not only the actors in the system but also the types of power they may have to exert influence. Power can be understood simply as the ability of one actor to shape the thinking and/or actions of other actors. At least eight types of power are at work in policy processes (Moon, 2019):

1. **Physical power:** The use of (or threat of) physical force to shape the thinking and action of others. An example of physical power is police officers enforcing a lockdown during a pandemic.
2. **Economic power:** The use of material resources to shape thinking and action. An example is the use of donor money to shape disease control priorities in a recipient country.
3. **Structural power:** The use of an actor's position in the social structure to wield influence. For example, a judge may use his or her structural power in a political system to block implementation of a law deemed unconstitutional.
4. **Institutional power:** The use of rules and decision-making procedures to shape thinking and action. For example, a civil society group may use its seat on the Board of the Global Fund to Fight AIDS, Tuberculosis and Malaria to influence the policies adopted by the organization.
5. **Moral power:** The ability to shape beliefs on right and wrong. Examples of moral power at work are "naming and shaming" strategies by advocates to convince powerful actors to change their policies or actions, such as when HIV/AIDS activists pressured multinational pharmaceutical companies to stop blocking the use of generic HIV medicines in low- and middle-income countries ('t Hoen et al., 2011).
6. **Discursive power:** The use of language and framing to shape how others understand an issue. For example, reframing an infectious disease as a security threat, rather than merely a public health issue, as happened with COVID-19, may mobilize money and political attention from new sources (though it may also have undesirable consequences such as sowing fear and panic) (McInnes and Lee, 2006).
7. **Power of expertise:** The ability to shape the legitimacy of knowledge, and therefore what is perceived as factually true. An example is the US Surgeon General's use of research to raise awareness of the harms of tobacco starting in the 1960s (Oreskes, 2010).
8. **Network power:** This refers to the use of personal relationships to wield influence. For example, the personal relationships built when business and political elites meet each year at the World Economic Forum in Davos can prove useful for future lobbying.

The latter four categories – moral, discursive, expertise and network power – may all fall under the broader category of what political scientist Joseph Nye has labeled "soft power" to distinguish it from "harder" military and economic power that has traditionally been seen to shape relations between nations.

Different actors have access to different forms of power to influence the policy process. For example, journalists have access to considerable discursive power, but not to physical power. Militaries have physical power, but may struggle to exert moral power. Religious leaders may have strong moral power, but little economic power.

Furthermore, these forms of power are often interrelated. To illustrate: an actor with significant financial resources (economic power), such as a self-made billionaire, can pay for a public relations firm to launch an advertising campaign to reframe an issue (discursive power) – for example, reframing personal gun ownership as a public health issue or, conversely, as an issue of personal freedom. This same billionaire may contribute to the election campaigns of several members of the US House of Representatives, and those representatives may then use their rights to propose and vote on legislation (institutional power) to promote or weaken gun control. The billionaire may also hire experts to write opinion pieces in newspapers or testify in legislative hearings (expert power) to support favored pieces of legislation or convince religious leaders (moral power) to make public statements in support of the proposed law. The combination of the institutional power of members of Congress, the power of experts and moral authorities and potential shifts in public opinion as a result of the advertising campaign could lead to the passage of a new law that would either facilitate or restrict gun ownership. This new law could then be enforced by the courts (structural power) and police forces (physical power). This example is hypothetical but is intended to illustrate how one type of power can be translated into another.

Many players interact in the policy process, each motivated by their own values and interests and each wielding various types of power to influence policy decisions. During the COVID-19 pandemic, we saw this typology at play across countries and stakeholders. Box 10.2 gives a few real-life examples that happened in 2020. Being able to identify who

Box 10.2 Different forms of power on display during the COVID-19 pandemic

- Physical power: The Philippines' police does house-to-house searches to force individuals with COVID-19 symptoms to get hospitalized (Lema and Morales, 2020).
- Economic power: Governments provide social safety nets, such as unemployment insurance and loans to businesses, to support those whose livelihoods are threatened.
- Structural power: Local authorities in cities issue reopening rules for bars and restaurants.
- Institutional power**:** The World Health Organization declares COVID-19 to comprise "a public health emergency of international concern" in January 2020, based on criteria governments agreed upon in the International Health Regulations (World Health Organization, 2020).
- Moral power: The Pope calls for greater international sharing of COVID-19 vaccines when they are in short supply.
- Discursive power: The United States president calls the coronavirus that caused COVID-19 the "Kung flu" virus (BBC, 2020).
- Power of expertise: The US Centers for Disease Control and Prevention recommends Americans to wear homemade cloth masks when industrially manufactured masks are in short supply (Adams, 2020).
- Network power: The leaders of the Global Alliance on Vaccines and Immunization (GAVI) and the Coalition for Epidemic Preparedness Innovations meet at a bar at the World Economic Forum's annual meeting in Davos, Switzerland, and come up with the idea that would later become COVAX, the global initiative that sought to supply COVID-19 vaccines to all countries equitably (Goldhill et al., 2021).

wields what kind of power is helpful to understand how policy processes get shaped and how social systems can change.

10.7 Theories of the Policy Process

Theories of the policy process can help make sense of the complexity of health system change. Among the many theories of policy processes, we highlight here two that are widely taught (Sabatier, 2007): the "multiple streams" framework developed by John Kingdon (Kingdon, 1993), and the advocacy coalition framework developed by Paul Sabatier and colleagues (Sabatier and Jenkins-Smith, 1988). While both frameworks were developed from the US domestic policy-making context, subsequent research has applied them productively to many other countries and the global level.

Kingdon's **multiple streams framework** (1984) conceptualizes the policy process as a complex system full of ambiguity. The views of key players are not necessarily known at a given time and may rapidly shift. Those with the discursive power to frame and reframe issues can therefore play a powerful role. Kingdon did not view policy-makers as rational actors with fixed interests or necessarily as holding clearly articulated positions, but rather as individuals with bounded rationality. Policy-makers face many competing demands on their time and will only pay attention to a problem if it is pressing or important enough.

Kingdon identified three mostly independent streams flowing through the policy system at any given time. First is the **problem stream**, which is the set of issues that stakeholders (e.g., voters, policy-makers, advocacy groups, business interests) want addressed in some way – in other words, they are the issues that have become problematized. An issue can come to be seen as a problem through the use of indicators (such as the number of new drug-resistant tuberculosis [DR-TB] cases globally in a given year), or crises or events (such as a sudden outbreak of TB). Second is the **policy stream**, which is the set of proposed solutions relevant to a given problem. Policies in this stream compete for attention and political backing but must be perceived as technically feasible and normatively acceptable to gain traction with policy-makers. In the previous DR-TB example, policies in the policy stream could include rolling out treatment programs for DR-TB, investing in an improved TB vaccine or screening at hospitals and clinics to identify patients with DR-TB. Finally, there is the **politics stream**, which could include changes in public opinion or the "national mood," turnover in the legislature or executive branch of government (e.g., after elections) or the impact of advocacy campaigns.

Kingdon argued that significant policy change is likely to occur when the three streams come together during time-limited **policy windows** during which time **policy entrepreneurs** proactively bring together the problem, policy and politics streams. A policy window can open because of a crisis (such as a sudden spike of an infectious disease) or a change in leadership (such as a new minister of health with certain priorities) and are usually short-lived. Policy entrepreneurs can be understood as individuals (or organizations) with the ability to make things happen when a policy window opens. They may sit in or outside government and may or may not be advocating for a particular solution. Their distinguishing feature is that they have adequate knowledge of the problem and potential solutions and can attract enough attention from overly busy decision-makers to effect change.

A second major theory of policy change is the **advocacy coalition framework** (ACF), initially developed by Sabatier and Jenkins-Smith in 1988 (Sabatier and Jenkins-Smith, 1988). The ACF posits that the technical complexity of most policy issues means that much of the policy-making process takes place within relatively small communities of specialists who form a **policy subsystem**. Examples of such subsystems might be those working on air pollution in the State of California, global vaccine production for pandemics, corruption in India's health care system or taxes on unhealthy foods in Massachusetts. Subsystems are usually delineated by a substantive issue area (e.g., air pollution) and a geographic territory (e.g., California). Furthermore, because actors in the system tend to maintain their values and hold stable beliefs, policy subsystems are relatively stable over time, with change processes often spanning a decade or more. In addition to the traditional recognition of law-makers, government agencies and interest groups as influential players in the policy process, the ACF emphasizes the role of information and therefore also focuses on journalists, researchers and analysts as key actors.

A policy subsystem may include hundreds of actors. In order to simplify and facilitate understanding of this complex system, the ACF proposes that such actors can be grouped into **advocacy coalitions** based on their values and policy positions. Thus, the key organizing principle of individuals in the policy subsystem is not necessarily their organizational affiliation, but rather the "deep core" and "policy core" beliefs that motivate each person. **Deep core beliefs** refer to fundamental philosophical values, such as the relative importance of collective versus individual rights, whereas **policy core beliefs** refer to beliefs relevant to a policy subsystem, such as the role of government intervention in the health insurance market. When actors with shared policy beliefs coordinate to achieve a certain policy, they form an advocacy coalition.

Because advocacy coalitions are relatively stable, significant policy change is generally caused by changes that are exogenous to the subsystem. Such shifts can include changes in the governing party, events in other subsystems, changes in the broader economy, the evolution of social norms or sudden shocks such as natural disasters. Nevertheless, internal shocks to the subsystem can also precipitate change and may include changes in key leadership when individuals retire, a major new source of financial backing for one coalition versus another or dramatic research findings by a coalition member that reframe the policy debate. Both external and internal changes can change the types and levels of power that actors wield within the policy subsystem, shifting the balance such that a dominant advocacy coalition becomes weaker or stronger, and is then able to change the policy status quo.

While both the multiple streams framework and ACF theories emphasize different factors, they are compatible with each other. Both emphasize that policy-making is a complex process, that significant change occurs infrequently (Baumgartner and Jones, 2010), that policy processes often play out over long time horizons and that endogenous or exogenous shocks to the system can create openings for change. Finally, while both frameworks recognize the constraints posed by structural factors, they also both recognize the importance and potential of individual agency to create lasting change.

What are the implications of these theories for this chapter's earlier discussion of health system dynamics? One is that health policy changes, such as increasing public financing of health care or expanding eligibility to new groups such as immigrants, do not happen steadily nor automatically. The multiple streams framework suggests such changes require policy entrepreneurs to seize the opportunity of a policy window, and to have readily at hand policy solutions to address an issue that has been successfully problematized. The ACF emphasizes that such health policy changes will occur when there is a shift in power between those who are for or against, for example, greater public health care financing or service provision to immigrants.

10.8 Summary

As we have seen in this chapter, health systems are dynamic.

The precise configuration of State involvement is a key feature to differentiate various types of health systems. Rather than classify health systems at the national level, we argue for using a lower level of aggregation – a modality. We used "modality" to refer to a particular configuration of State involvement in stewardship, financing and delivery of health services based on a specific principle for population eligibility, that is, purchasing power, poverty, socially perceived priority and citizenship.

In the past, many health systems were organized by population groups, but more recently many nations have been trying to organize their health systems by functions rather than by population groups. The five essential health system functions (stewardship, systemic integration, financing, service provision and resource generation) are performed for the population as a whole. We hypothesize that many health systems have evolved along a trajectory over which the State gradually increases its degree of control, notably over the stewardship and financing functions, while an increasing proportion of the population is covered by the health system.

Significant changes in health systems are political processes often involving many types of actors wielding different forms of power. Health policy change usually takes place in a pattern of punctuated equilibrium, a result of purposeful efforts, windows of opportunity and in a context of political contestation.

In Chapter 11, we examine common challenges hindering health system reform.

Comprehension and Discussion Questions

- Think of a country you know well, then describe the role the government plays in the health system. Which functions does it perform (e.g., stewardship, financing and/or service provision)? Which social groups are eligible to receive which services (e.g., formal sector workers, older adults, children, low-income government employees)?
- Think about a recent health topic in your country. Identify at least three different types of power that influence how that health topic is addressed, based on the typology in this chapter. Which actors use which type(s) of power?
- What is a recent example of a policy window?
- Sabatier distinguishes between deep core beliefs and policy core beliefs. What is the difference between the two concepts? What is an example of each?

Papers from Which This Chapter Is Adapted

Frenk, J. 1994. Dimensions of health system reform. *Health Policy*, 27, 19–34.

Frenk, J. 2015. Leading the way towards universal health coverage: a call to action. *The Lancet*, 385, 1352–1358.

Frenk, J. & Donabedian, A. 1987. State intervention in medical care: types, trends and variables. *Health Policy and Planning*, 2, 17–31.

Kingdon, J. 1993. *Agendas, Alternatives and Public Policies.* New York: Harper Collins.

Moon, S. 2019. Power in global governance: an expanded typology from global health. *Globalization and Health*, 15, 74.

Sabatier, P. (ed.) 2007. *Theories of the Policy Process.* Cambridge, MA: Westview Press.

Chapter 11 Challenges of Health System Reform

Learning Objectives

- Define health system reform, distinguishing between four different levels of change: systemic, programmatic, organizational and instrumental.
- Identify the main challenges facing reform efforts for each of the five functions of health systems (financing, provision of services, resource generation, stewardship and systemic integration).
- Understand the different functions of health systems, how they can be reformed and associated challenges through an extended case study of the 2003 Seguro Popular reform in Mexico.

11.1 Introduction

As mentioned in Chapter 9, comparative studies reveal huge heterogeneity in the performance of different health systems. There is wide variation in the health indicators of countries with similar levels of income per capita that spend similar amounts of money on their respective health systems (World Bank, 1993).

Because of this variation, there is an almost universal search for better ways of regulating, financing and delivering health services. As pointed out in Chapter 9, the search is being undertaken with equal intensity in countries at all levels of economic development and with all types of political regimes. Finding better answers to the new economic, social and epidemiological realities is the challenge of health system reform.

In this chapter, we first look at the various policy levels where reform can take place. We then examine the general characteristics of such reforms and the challenges facing efforts to improve the various health system functions. In the final part, we illustrate these characteristics and challenges through a case study of the 2003 Mexican health reform, whose main innovation was a public insurance program called Seguro Popular.

11.2 Health System Reform: Policy Levels

In the health field, as in many other areas of human endeavor, the term "reform" has been given multiple meanings, sometimes in an attempt to lend legitimacy to a particular set of actions. This is not surprising, since reform has a positive connotation, as it is usually associated with the removal of negative elements or the willed evolution toward better stages of being. In contrast to revolution, reform is meant to be an incremental and peaceful change. More specifically, health system reform can be defined as "changes produced out of explicit intention on the part of government or political groups to

Table 11.1 Health system reform: policy levels

Policy level	Main objective	Issues
Systemic	Equity	Basis for population eligibility Institutional arrangements: • Public agencies involved in health care • Levels of government • Public/private mix • Population involvement • Resource generators • Other sectors with effects on health
Programmatic	Allocational efficiency	Priority setting Cost-effectiveness of interventions
Organizational	Technical efficiency	Productivity Quality of care
Instrumental	Institutional intelligence for performance improvement	Information systems Scientific research Technological development Human resource development

transform, for the better, the health sector" (Frenk and González-Block, 1992). Berman proposes that the essence of reform is "sustained, purposeful change to improve the efficiency, equity, and effectiveness of the health sector" (Berman, 1993).

If we wish to better understand the nature of health system reforms, it is useful to consider that there are four major levels of health policy: systemic, programmatic, organizational and instrumental. The main objectives of each level, as well as the issues it deals with, are summarized in Table 11.1. Any health system reform addresses these issues to meet the respective objectives.

Simply stated, the **systemic** level deals with the roles and responsibilities of the main actors that constitute the health system, as identified in Chapter 7. Hence, the major issues refer both to the adoption of a principle for population eligibility and to the institutional arrangements specifying the public agencies involved in health care, the distribution of functions between central and local government, the public/private mix, the degree and forms of population involvement, the relationship with resource generators and the principles and relationships governing the broader system of health. Equity should be the guiding objective of reform efforts at this level, although we observe that may not always be the case, for example, when criteria for population eligibility change to exclude certain groups (undocumented migrants, for example).

Having specified, at the systemic level, the basic structure of health care in a country, policy must then define the content in terms of actual programs and interventions. Hence, the main objective of the **programmatic** level is allocational efficiency, through an explicit consideration of priorities by criteria such as cost-effectiveness of interventions and social acceptability (Jamison et al., 1993). A major exercise of health system

Table 11.2 Change in health systems

Policy level	Type of change	
Systemic	Restructure or redesign	REFORM
Programmatic	Reorientation or reprogramming	
Organizational	Reorganization	
Instrumental	Reinforcement	

reform at this level is to define a package of cost-effective interventions that can be made universally available.

Regardless of what interventions are included in the package, it is necessary for policy to move into the actual organizations that produce services. Even if an allocationally efficient set of interventions is produced by the health system, the **organizational** level must still assure technical efficiency by looking at the issues of productivity and quality.

Crossing across the three foregoing levels is a set of **instrumental** policies, which are intended to generate the institutional intelligence required for better system performance. Such intelligence takes form in information systems, scientific research, technological innovation and human resource development.

The advantage of dividing health policy into the four proposed levels is that it prevents us from adopting an "all or nothing" view of reform efforts. Thus, if there is political resistance to change at one level, it is still possible to make progress at the other levels. Yet, it should be realized that the four policy levels are profoundly interrelated, so that a comprehensive reform strategy must contemplate all of them. In fact, it could be proposed, as shown in Table 11.2, that partial changes at each level are different from full-fledged reform. Thus, when only the systemic level is transformed, we can speak of restructuring or redesign. Similarly, efforts at altering the substantive priorities of the health system constitute reorientation or reprogramming. A country may also engage in reorganization when it restricts its change efforts to improving the quality and efficiency of the actual production of services. Finally, when the instrumental level is the focus of change, we can speak of reinforcement. The message, then, is clear: Any of these four types of change can be, in and of itself, a valuable step forward, but a true reform must address all of them, paying close attention to their mutual interrelations. This is the concept of reform that is consistent with the broad goal of accelerating the health system transition we discussed in Chapter 9.

The foregoing proposal should not be seen as a mere conceptual or semantic exercise. Its main purpose is to serve as a framework that policy-makers can use in specifying the full array of elements that are potentially open to reform, so that they can lay out, in a clear way, the options for improving the health system.

11.3 Characteristics of Reform

In Chapter 9, we explored the limitations of current models of organizing health systems and the dynamics through which a new model seems to be emerging in the ongoing generation of health system reforms. Here are some of the attributes of this emerging model.

The first characteristic of such reforms is the **organization of health systems by functions** (Figure 10.2). The transition to this type of organization has been moving forward, but at an uneven pace and with some reversals, as we will illustrate below with the case of Mexico.

A second characteristic of the emerging model, strongly associated with the idea of overcoming health system segmentation and social segregation, is the **change in eligibility rules**. Universal health coverage is increasingly grounded in the idea that traditional social insurance schemes have excluded large sectors of the population (especially the self-employed and unemployed), thus reproducing social inequality by leaving people with lower income further behind. In a growing number of countries, the protection of health is now recognized as a universal social right and is being gradually de-linked from formal employment and labor market status (Atun et al., 2015; Yamin and Frisancho, 2015).

A third component of this model is the **emphasis on explicit entitlements**, which adopt the form of covered interventions, such as those included in the Mandatory Health Plan in Colombia, the Universal Catalog of Essential Health Services of Seguro Popular in Mexico, the AUGE program in Chile, the Universal Coverage Scheme in Thailand and the Health Benefit Package Policy in Malawi. As mentioned earlier, the constitutions of many countries include rights, principles and standards related to health, but have often lacked a legal definition of the entitlements that ensue from them. According to Brachet-Márquez (2001), the transformation of health care into a social right requires the definition of the set of interventions that all citizens, regardless of their labor or socio-economic status, should receive and can legally demand.

Packages of health services were designed originally as priority-setting tools for resource-constrained settings. Cost-effectiveness analysis has been used to identify those interventions that generate the largest benefits for the available public resources. Usually, these essential services have been provided to people with lower incomes. In some recent reforms (such as in our case study for Mexico), intervention packages have still responded to priority-setting concerns, but they have also been used as a planning and quality assurance tool, and as a core component of a universalistic conception of coverage that requires the explicit definition of benefits (Frenk and Gómez-Dantés, 2009). As a planning instrument, these packages have been used to estimate the resources needed to strengthen health systems. As a quality assurance tool, they have been adopted to make sure that all necessary services are provided following standardized protocols. Finally, and most importantly, these packages have also been used to empower health care users by making them aware of their entitlements.

The fourth characteristic of the emerging model is the **expanded scope of health reforms** associated with it. Many reforms implemented in the second half of the past century were designed around specific delivery interventions targeted mostly at maternal and child health. The new reforms implemented are broader in three senses: (i) they move beyond the delivery function to also address challenges related to stewardship and financing; (ii) they include initiatives to deal not only with the unfinished agenda but also with non-communicable diseases and injuries; and (iii) they expand the scope of health systems to include comprehensive health care services, public health programs (such as pandemic preparedness and response) and interventions to address upstream social determinants of health.

The final characteristic, which underlies the previous ones, is an explicit discussion of the **ethical basis of reform**. The starting premise for this ethical pillar is that every health system reflects value assumptions, which are expressed in the distribution of benefits and the organization of its institutions. For example, the 2003 Mexican reform was formulated and promoted on the basis of a guiding concept and a set of explicit values, which are related to the principle that health care is not a commodity or a privilege, but a social right. Thus, the guiding concept was the "democratization of health." The term democratization implies "the application of the norms and procedures of citizenship to those institutions that have been governed by other principles, such as coercive control, social tradition, judgment of specialists, or bureaucratic processes" (O'Donnel and Schmitter, 1991). The term "citizen" is used in a broad sense to include all the persons legally residing in a country. This concept is related to a range of rights and duties as defined within a constitution (Scruton, 1996). In his seminal work, Thomas Humphrey Marshall recognizes three types of rights involved in the idea of citizenship: civil, political and social (Marshall, 1965). According to him, citizenship culminates in the effective exercise of social rights.

In addition to this guiding concept, five values related to it were adopted by the Mexican reform (Frenk, 2006):

- **Social inclusion:** This is based on the premise that all human lives have the same value and that health systems must represent instances in which everybody receives similar treatment for similar needs.
- **Equal opportunity:** This postulates that distribution of wealth can only be considered fair if each generation enters life with the same opportunities, which are largely determined by public health interventions addressing the social determinants of health and by access to high-quality health services.
- **Financial justice:** This means that individuals contribute to the health system according to their economic capacity and receive services according to their health needs, in such a way that a large enough risk pool is aggregated to facilitate three types of solidarity: risk solidarity (between the healthy and the sick), generational solidarity (between the young and the old) and distributive solidarity (between those with more or less wealth).
- **Individual autonomy:** This means that every person enjoys the freedom to decide what is more appropriate for him or her, a prerogative that the family unit assumes in the case of minors and of people with limitations in their capabilities to decide.
- **Social responsibility:** This places limits on the freedom proposed by the previous value, specifically on the freedom to be neglectful of one's own health in a way that puts other persons at risk. Additionally, the involuntary nature of most health deficits imposes a shared responsibility to care for the individuals who experience them. The tension between individual autonomy and social responsibility was made explicit during the COVID-19 pandemic around the sometimes acrimonious debates on the required use of face masks.

Guided by an explicit ethical framework, many countries have embarked on actual processes of reform. We will next explore the challenges faced by those initiatives.

11.4 Challenges of Change

We analyze the main challenges by looking at the crucial functions of the health system. Figure 7.3, which was introduced in Chapter 7, summarizes those functions: financing (including its three subfunctions of revenue collection, fund pooling and purchasing), provision of both personal and non-personal services, resource generation, stewardship and systemic integration. We also analyze how in every health system in the world, there is a public–private mix. Typically, we recognize that stewardship is a quintessential public function, because it involves setting the rules of the game, providing strategic direction and assessing performance. Similarly, systemic integration involves public policies and programs in other systems that affect the social determinants of health. Most finance should be public, although in every country there is some degree of private financing, through private insurance, other prepayment schemes or out-of-pocket payments, which still account for the largest share of expenditures in many low- and middle-income countries. Private participation further increases when it comes to service provision and resource generation. Getting this mix right is probably the single most complex and pervasive policy question. A functional analysis can be a very powerful tool to diagnose and improve health systems, whether they are local, national or global.

11.4.1 Challenges of Financing

Many health systems segment families according to their occupational status, excluding the self-employed and unemployed populations from insurance coverage. That is why many reform initiatives, including Obamacare in the United States and Seguro Popular in Mexico, sought to make access to health insurance independent of a person's position in the labor market.

A major financial challenge in segmented health systems is the fragmentation of the risk pool, which weakens the three types of solidarity we described before: risk solidarity (between the healthy and the sick), generational solidarity (between the young and the old) and socioeconomic solidarity (between those with more or less wealth). The whole idea of insurance is that you contribute when you are healthy, so that when you are sick, you can be treated without further payment. Healthy people can work and generate income. That is the time to pay for care, either through taxes or premiums. Sick people cannot work and are vulnerable, so out-of-pocket payments are very inefficient. Regardless of wealth, everyone will at one point benefit from the risk solidarity that lies at the core of universal health insurance. That is why it is so compelling as a matter of social policy and why it is such a common feature of reform efforts aimed at expanding the risk pool.

The most common challenge of the purchasing subfunction refers to the definition of priorities regarding which services will be paid for, since no health system, even in the wealthiest countries, can cover every medically useful procedure. Often, countries lack transparent, defensible mechanisms for priority setting. The absence of clear priorities leads to allocational inefficiency. When you do not have clear rules for priority setting, you end up with inertial budgeting and unstructured purchasing.

11.4.2 Challenges of Health Service Provision

Health service provision is where the population and the providers come together. Each plays multiple roles, as we have seen, and there are many potential mismatches: there are huge information asymmetries; very different expectations on the part of the two; and different incentives. At the extreme, when providers get paid through fee-for-service they have an incentive to increase the volume of services, which may not be exactly what the population needs or wants. A further challenge refers to heterogeneity in several dimensions, like the price per procedure and the quality of care.

11.4.3 Challenges of Resource Generation

In resource generation, the big problem is the balance between patients' health needs, the capacity to translate a need into demand for services and the supply of resources. A good health system is one that aligns health needs, service demand and resource supply. Such a system generates enough resources – human, technological and informational – to provide high-quality services that meet the health needs and expectations of a population. That, we would say, is a harmonious or balanced health system.

11.4.4 Challenges of Stewardship

Looking around the world, there is typically weak capacity in ministries of health to carry out the stewardship function in an effective, efficient and transparent way. Many ministries still devote most of their resources and attention to the direct delivery of services, principally to people with lesser means in their country – a very important function, but one that can be carried out by other actors in a decentralized manner. Such ministries tend to have low capacity for regulation and strategic design of the system. Very often, the regulations are rigid, ineffective and prone to corruption. If we look around the world, especially in low- and middle-income countries, most do not accredit facilities, and do not have expeditious and efficient procedures for licensing providers. They face major problems assuring the quality of inputs, like drugs.

11.4.5 Challenges of Systemic Integration

Challenges related to systemic integration are perhaps the most complex of all, in part because the factors driving this function are still emerging from the interconnected social, economic and environmental crises magnified by the COVID-19 pandemic.

First, determinants further away from individual health, while having enormous potential, are also the hardest to track in terms of causal pathways. In other words, it is difficult to draw causal relationships from a change in a structural or societal determinant and a change in health outcomes.

Second, collaboration among different parts of a government is often not well aligned with the way governments operate in terms of planning, policy design and implementation. For example, budgets might not be easily fungible across sectors. Public servants might not easily pivot their focus to new goals. It is not surprising that most Health in All Policies experiments have happened in high-income countries, such as Finland, Norway and Australia, which often bolster strong government agencies with sophisticated processes and advanced data systems (Greszczuk, 2019). Most governments might not be well equipped to implement the type of flexible, highly fungible processes required for a true whole-of-government approach.

Finally, collaboration is hard. Power dynamics, along with personal or institutional interests, may often get in the way of successful multi-actor coordination. For example, a recent study by Hagen et al. (2018) found a negative relationship between the employment of public health coordinators in Norwegian municipalities and prioritizing fair distribution of social and economic resources among social groups in local health promotion initiatives. Other authors have linked this result to the risk of Health in All Policies efforts being perceived by other sectors as "health imperialism," which generates resistance to integration efforts (Delaney et al., 2016; Holt and Ahlmark, 2018). Amidst these challenges, the World Health Organization has compiled and analyzed successful case stories of multisectoral and intersectoral initiatives in various countries to share best practices to improve health and well-being through collaboration around the world (World Health Organization, 2018).

11.5 Innovations by Function: A Case Study

Despite these hurdles, many health challenges are being met. The reform movement that began in the 1990s, accelerated in the 2010s with the global movement for universal health coverage. Mexico offers a relevant case study of using the five functions framework to design specific innovations, as summarized in Figure 11.1.

A series of studies carried out in Mexico during the late 1990s identified disturbing rates of catastrophic health expenditures (Frenk, 1995). Such a critical situation was due to the fact that approximately half of the Mexican population, 50 million people then, lacked health insurance. The analysis exposed a dreadful paradox: we know that health contributes to the reduction of poverty, yet medical care can itself produce financial stress when a country lacks the social instruments to assure fair financing of personal health care services.

In 2003, the federal government secured support from all political parties for legislation aimed at correcting that paradox. A reform to the National Health Law created the System for Social Protection in Health (SSPH). The most prominent component of SSPH was Seguro Popular, a public insurance scheme which provided social protection in health to the population without social security.

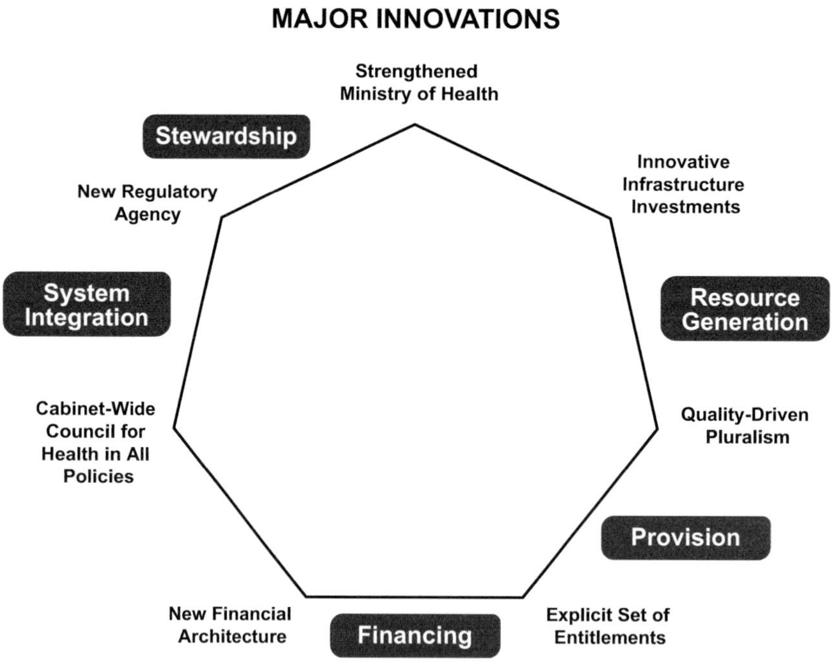

Figure 11.1 Major policy innovations by health system function in Mexico.

11.5.1 Financing

We first turn our attention to the first function of health systems: health financing.

11.5.1.1 New Financial Architecture

Seguro Popular began implementation on January 1, 2004. It was funded predominantly through federal and state subsidies, and guaranteed access to a package of essential services provided in ambulatory settings and general hospitals, as well as a package of high-cost interventions, financed through a special fund (Fund for Protection against Catastrophic Health Expenditures) and provided by national and regional high-specialty hospitals. Public expenditure was gradually expanded to finance comprehensive health care coverage for those excluded from conventional, employment-based social insurance. By 2018, over 53 million people were enrolled in the new scheme, and the budget of the Ministry of Health had been multiplied four times in real terms (i.e., adjusting for inflation).

The new funding model implied an important change in incentives for state governments and providers. Funding for each state was determined largely by the number of individuals affiliated to Seguro Popular and was thus driven by demand. Enrollment was voluntary, yet the reform also included incentives for expanding coverage. States had an incentive to affiliate the entire population, since their budgets were determined by an annual, per capita allocation. The voluntary nature of the affiliation was a key component of the process, since it offered incentives for quality and efficiency: if states provided wasteful care, the money they received would not be enough to meet the demand, but if quality was low, individuals would not re-affiliate.

11.5.1.2 Explicit Set of Entitlements

Two key instruments of the reform were the package of essential services and the package of high-cost interventions, both of which were legally mandated. By 2018, Seguro Popular affiliates had guaranteed access to 290 essential services and 65 high-cost interventions, including neonatal intensive care and treatment for all cancers in children, cervical and breast cancer and HIV/AIDS, among others. The process of defining the high-cost interventions was dynamic. The law stipulated that the package would be expanded and updated periodically based on changes in the epidemiological profile, technological developments and the availability of resources. The covered services were selected using cost-effectiveness analyses and ethical deliberations on social acceptability criteria. Apart from serving as a priority-setting tool, the notion of a package of interventions was also a means of empowering people by making entitlements explicit.

11.5.2 Provision: Quality-Driven Delivery

In addition to the incentives implicit in the Seguro Popular enrollment mechanism, the Mexican reform developed an explicit system-wide strategy to promote quality of health care. Its vision was to convert quality into a core value of the national health system, including both public and private providers, in a pluralistic framework with common requirements and standards. Its three main objectives were to improve specific quality metrics, reduce variation among states and institutions, and improve public perceptions on the quality of services. The main components of this strategy were the training of providers on quality of care; the accreditation of public and private health care organizations; and the monitoring of quality of care as the driver of a continuous improvement strategy.

11.5.3 Resource Generation: Innovative Infrastructure Investments

The Mexican health reform included a Master Plan for Investment in Infrastructure designed to expand the availability and capacity of health care facilities, including ambulatory units and general and specialized hospitals. To maximize efficiency, funding for new facilities was determined on the basis of a needs assessment undertaken by the Ministry of Health in all locations. By 2011, around 2,000 outpatient units, 200 general hospitals and 15 high-specialty regional hospitals had been built.

A complement to the plan in infrastructure was the corresponding Master Plan for Investment in Medical Equipment, designed and implemented by an office also created during the reform years, the National Center for Excellence in Health Technology. This plan established robust maintenance procedures for medical equipment and rationalized the adoption of new technology through evidence-based analyses and needs assessments.

11.5.4 Stewardship: Strengthened Ministry of Health

One of the initial measures of the Mexican health reform was to reinforce the stewardship capacities of the Ministry of Health, including strategic planning, monitoring and evaluation. These activities were based on the intensive use of evidence and information, gathered by a modernized National Health Information System, which included regular registration subsystems and periodical national health surveys. Information and monitoring systems were used, among other things, to assure transparency in the allocation of resources and to monitor service utilization, quality of care and health outcomes. An important innovation was the creation of a comprehensive evaluation system with three components: (i) monitoring of personal and public health services; (ii) program evaluation; and (iii) health system performance assessment. The assumption behind this framework was that the first component would be useful mostly for management, the third mostly for policy, and the second for both, bearing in mind that all three components would be crucial for accountability purposes. Through the program evaluation component, an external evaluation of Seguro Popular, using a quasi-experimental design, was carried out. This evaluation is considered one of the largest randomized health policy experiments ever. Its main finding was a reduction in catastrophic expenditures attributable to Seguro Popular (King et al., 2009).

11.5.5 Systemic Integration

Finally, the reform addressed the last function of our health system framework: systemic integration, that is, the relationships between the health system and other systems.

11.5.5.1 New Regulatory Agency

In 2001, a new regulatory agency, the Federal Commission for Protection against Health Risks (COFEPRIS), was created. This commission is responsible for food safety, definition of environmental standards, promotion of occupational safety and prevention of work-related injury, regulation of the pharmaceutical industry and control of hazardous substances like alcohol, tobacco and sugar-sweetened beverages (SSBs). This agency has played a crucial role in the design and implementation of policies to combat tobacco consumption, which include cigarette excise taxes, health warnings, smoke-free air laws and marketing restrictions. Thanks to these measures, Mexico was one of the four countries in the world that were able to reduce smoking prevalence in the population aged 15 years or older by half between 1980 and 2012. COFEPRIS has also played an important role in the successful implementation of SSB taxes in Mexico.

11.5.5.2 Cabinet-Wide Council for Health in All Policies

A constitutional body called the General Health Council was transformed into an inclusive entity to coordinate other cabinet departments around specific policies designed to advance health as a shared objective of the entire government. In addition to the aforementioned fiscal policy to reduce consumption of tobacco and SSBs, a salient example was the close coordination with the ministries of social development and of education in a successful conditional cash transfer targeted to low-income families, which has been extensively evaluated and adapted by other countries (World Bank, 2014).

11.6 Policy Transitions

Figure 11.2 summarizes a set of key policy transitions that have characterized recent reform experiences in many countries, including the Mexican case: from rigid regulation to strategic stewardship; from fragmented revenue collection to prepayment based on solidarity; from limited fund pooling to broad fund pooling based on sound actuarial principles for optimal risk management; from inertial unstructured purchasing to active purchasing based on clear priorities; from heterogeneous provision in terms of cost and quality to quality-driven provision; from imbalanced resource generation to balanced resource generation. Ultimately, the largest change, the true paradigm shift, is to move from a health system that segments the population into groups with different rights to a health system that separates functions while providing universal coverage with equal rights.

11.7 Political Sustainability

As discussed in Chapter 10, health system reforms are a function of the policy processes and power dynamics in place within the broader political system. Seguro Popular is no

Rigid Regulation	→	**Strategic Stewardship**
Fragmented Revenue Collection	→	**Solidarity-Based Prepayment**
Limited Fund Pooling	→	**Broad Fund Pooling**
Inertial and Unstructured Purchasing	→	**Active Purchasing**
Heterogeneous Provision	→	**Quality-Driven Provision**
Imbalanced Resource Generation	→	**Balanced Resource Generation**
Segmentation of Population Groups	→	**Separation of Functions**

Figure 11.2 Key policy transitions.

exception and provides an apt illustration of Kingdon's multiple streams framework introduced in Chapter 9. For decades, those who were formally employed in the private sector or by the government received health insurance coverage in a corporatist model that segmented the population based on employment status. However, half the population was uninsured, which meant many lacked access to care, and households faced high costs, as described earlier, which provided a compelling **problem stream**. Policy experts had proposed overhauling the system to expand coverage, forming a **policy stream**. However, it was only after Mexico's historic presidential election of 2000 – the first fully democratic election in 72 years – that a window of opportunity opened to launch an ambitious reform. Following the election, the new government needed to find ways to legitimize and consolidate its rule, so it recruited a technically competent team to develop evidence-based policy proposals for health reform, which strengthened the policy stream. Finally, by delegating key decision-making authority to the states while increasing the financial resources they would receive from the federal government, the reform was structured to mobilize political support from state governors to overcome opposition from both those resistant to changing the status quo and those who felt the reform did not go far enough, providing a way forward for the **politics stream**. As mentioned earlier, ultimately the legislative changes that underpinned the reform were agreed to by all parties, and the implementation process involved every state in the country. In other words, the problem, policy and politics streams came together during the window of opportunity opened by the transition to democracy, allowing for significant health system reform to be approved and implemented. Opposition to the reforms did not disappear, however, as explained below.

In addition, Seguro Popular has been one of the most thoroughly studied programs in the world through the comprehensive evaluation framework described earlier under innovations in the stewardship function. A thorough literature review (Knaul et al., 2012) published eight years after large-scale implementation of Seguro Popular identified over 100 peer-reviewed articles, including the randomized assessments mentioned above. The evidence overwhelmingly points to major benefits in terms of financial protection, effective coverage of health services and improved health status, without inducing any significant distortion in the labor market. Based on such evidence, the influential publication *The Economist* hailed this reform as an exemplary model for achieving universal health coverage: "Studies suggest that Seguro Popular has drastically reduced the number of Mexicans facing catastrophic health costs and reduced infant mortality" (The Economist, 2018).

Largely because of the positive evidence stemming from rigorous evaluations, Seguro Popular continued to receive strong policy and financial support from the two presidential administrations following the one in which it was created. Since in Mexico presidents are elected for a single six-year term, this meant that over almost two decades Seguro Popular drove the largest expansion of population coverage, health care infrastructure and budgets in the history of the country.

Yet, in 2018 Mexican citizens elected a populist president, as part of a larger wave of populism that had affected many parts of the world. Some of the defining characteristics of populism include a distrust of technical expertise, a tendency to base policy on ideological preconceptions rather than scientific evidence and a claim that the previous status quo must be superseded through the authoritarian will of the leader. In terms of

Sabatier's advocacy coalition framework, this was an external shock, which shifted the power balance between two competing coalitions, one that favored Seguro Popular and the other that sought different policy approaches to the organization of the health system. It was not surprising, therefore, that, along with serious reversals in many other policy domains, the new populist government in Mexico decided to cancel Seguro Popular, regressing to the segmented structure that had characterized the health system before the reform. The timing of this decision was unfortunate, since its implementation coincided with the start of the COVID-19 pandemic. The ensuing disruption in the operations of the health system is part of the reason why Mexico had one of the least effective responses to the pandemic (UCSF Institute for Global Health Sciences, 2021). In addition, there has been a loss of coverage, an increase in catastrophic expenditures and a reversal in critical indicators like maternal mortality and life expectancy (Knaul et al., 2023).

Clearly, various problems had accumulated after almost 20 years of extensive and intensive implementation of Seguro Popular, especially heterogeneous performance among different states in a federal system, as well as isolated yet scandalous incidents of corruption after years of budgetary growth. To surmount these challenges, there was and still is ample room for bold reform initiatives, most importantly to overcome the segmentation between Seguro Popular and conventional social insurance, so that Mexico can advance toward a truly universal health system.

Most importantly, the dismantling of Seguro Popular illustrates the fact that progress in health policy is not linear but can experience reversals. Some may believe that improvements brought about by enlightened policies are self-preserving because they have proven their worth in ways that guard them against biased and narrow-minded attacks. This is not the case. Societies should not underestimate how policy changes can suddenly occur in patterns of punctuated equilibrium. No matter how well they perform, we should never take programs or institutions for granted (Frenk et al., 2019).

11.8 Summary

In this chapter, we defined health system reform as "changes produced out of explicit intention on the part of government or political groups to transform, for the better, the health sector." We identified four levels where such changes could be made: systemic (dealing with the roles and responsibilities of the main actors that constitute the health system), where the main goal is equity; programmatic, where the main objective is allocational efficiency; organizational, where the objective is technical efficiency; and instrumental, where institutional intelligence is developed for better system performance. Valuable change can happen at any of these four levels, but true reform must address all of them, paying close attention to their mutual interrelations. We examined reform challenges in each of the five health system functions – financing, provision of services, resource generation, stewardship and systemic integration – as well as innovations within them. Finally, we analyzed several key policy transitions and larger societal transformations that are shaping the future of health systems. We concluded by using the case of Mexico to illustrate how these ideas came together in the actual design and implementation of comprehensive health system reform.

In Chapter 12, we extend our analysis of national health systems to the global level.

Comprehension and Discussion Questions

- In this chapter, we propose four levels of health policy reforms: systemic, programmatic, organizational and instrumental. What is the objective of each level? What type of reforms could each level entail?
- Choose one function of a health system and describe the challenges that may arise when reforming this function.
- Describe the three streams and the policy window of the Kingdon model (from Chapter 10), using either the Mexican reform discussed in this chapter or a health reform you are familiar with.

Papers from Which This Chapter Is Adapted

Frenk, J. 2014. Leading the way towards universal health coverage: a call to action. *The Lancet*, 385, 1352–1358.

Frenk, J. & Gómez-Dantés, O. 2009. Ideas and ideals: ethical basis of health reform in Mexico. *The Lancet*, 373, 1406–1408.

For the case study on the Mexican health reform, a comprehensive review of the literature about this experience can be found in the following:

Knaul, F. M., González-Pier, E., Gómez-Dantés, O. et al. 2012. The quest for universal health coverage: achieving social protection for all in Mexico. *The Lancet*, 380, 1259–1279.

Chapter 12 The Global Health System: Extending the Organized Social Response

Learning Objectives

- Define the global health system, including its main actors and its boundaries.
- Describe three types of governance challenges that currently impede the global health system: the sovereignty challenge, the sectoral challenge and the accountability challenge.
- Identify the essential functions of the global health system.
- Discuss current challenges and barriers to establish a better functioning global health system.

12.1 Introduction

Just as the national health system is the organized social response to health conditions at the national level, the global health system can be conceptualized as the organized social response to the cross-border transfer of health risks. As detailed in Chapter 2, globalization has intensified the health risks (and opportunities) brought on by the movement of people, goods, services, ideas and rules across borders, as so clearly illustrated by the COVID-19 pandemic (see Chapter 14).

The global health system can be defined as the group of actors in the global public domain whose primary intent is to improve health, along with the rules and norms governing their interactions (Szlezák et al., 2010). At the core of the system are national governments, with their specialized health ministries, departments or agencies and, in the case of donor nations, the health programs of their respective bilateral development cooperation agencies. National governments coordinate their responses to common health challenges through a variety of mechanisms, such as regional organizations like the European Union (EU) or Association of Southeast Asian Nations.

The World Health Organization (WHO) is the only actor in the global health system that is built on the near-universal membership of all United Nations member states (though it is often identified only with its secretariat), and it therefore is central to the system. Also important to the system are other United Nations and multilateral agencies that have health components (e.g., the United Nations Children's Fund known by its acronym UNICEF, the World Bank and the regional development banks), along with a diverse set of civil society organizations, multinational corporations, foundations, traditional and social media, religious groups, professional organizations and academic institutions – among others. This pluralistic landscape has been enriched by a set of innovative and influential hybrid organizations, such as the GAVI Alliance (formerly the Global Alliance for Vaccines and Immunization), UNITAID (which works to improve the functioning of global markets for health products for its priority diseases), and the Global Fund to Fight AIDS, Tuberculosis and Malaria, all of which are governed by representatives both from within and from outside national governments – hence the term "hybrid." To make matters even more complex, health is increasingly influenced by decisions that are made in other global policy-making arenas, such as those governing international trade, security, agriculture and the environment (Smith, 2006; Costello et al., 2009; Lee et al., 2009b).

In this chapter, we first explore three key challenges faced by the global health system today: the sovereignty challenge, the sectorial challenge and the accountability challenge. We then propose four functions of an effective global health system. Finally, we discuss governance of the overall system and the current barriers to establishing a better functioning global system.

12.2 Governance Challenges in Global Health

Actors in the global policy arenas illustrated in Figure 12.1 influence health, even though that is not their primary intent. A major example of such an institution is the World Trade Organization, which has profoundly shaped domestic and global intellectual property rules relating to pharmaceuticals, among other health-related trade issues.

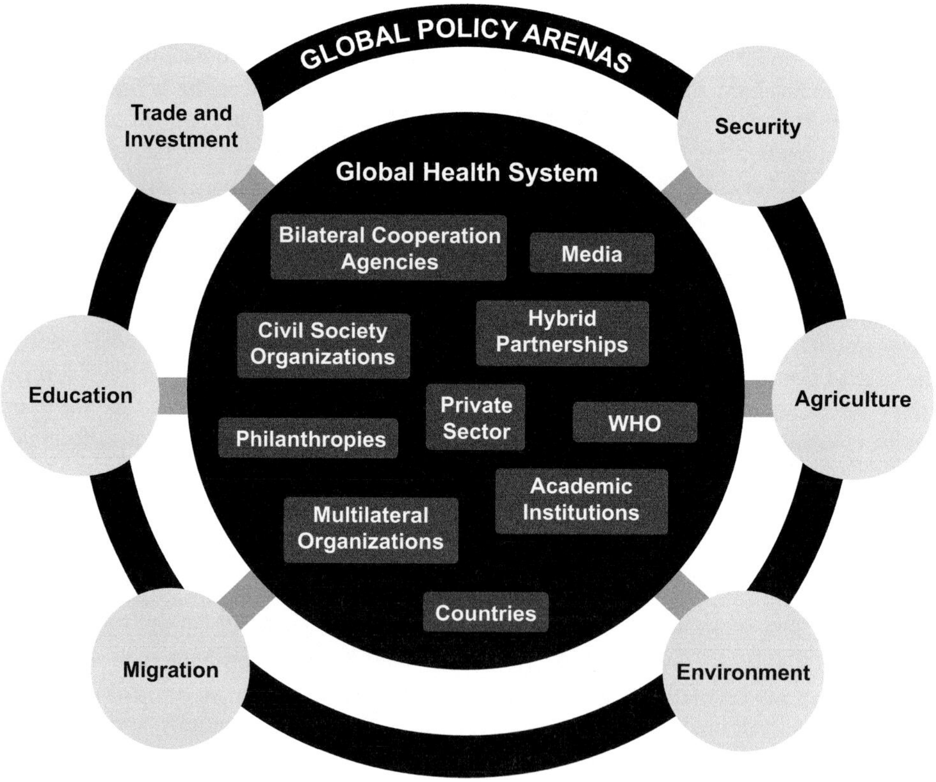

Figure 12.1 The global health system. Adapted from Frenk, J. & Moon, S. (2013). Governance challenges in global health. *The New England Journal of Medicine*, 368(10), 936–942.

These policy-making institutions are not part of the global health system; instead, they represent critical policy arenas in which global health actors must learn to exert influence. The importance of these arenas is the reason why we prefer the term "global governance for health," rather than the more restrictive notion of "global health governance," which tends to focus only on governance of the global health system (the inner circle in Figure 12.1) (Lee et al., 2009a; Lee and Kamradt-Scott; 2014; Moon, 2018).

The challenge of governing the diverse group of actors within the global health system has drawn increased political attention (Fidler, 2007; Lee and Fidler, 2007; Fidler, 2010; Moon et al., 2010; Bloom, 2011). Thus far, however, too little attention has been given to the problem of protecting and promoting health in governance processes outside the global health system (Ottersen et al., 2014). "Good" global governance for health should exhibit at least the following key traits: effectiveness, equity and efficiency in achieving outcomes, as well as legitimacy in decision-making processes. However, the achievement of these goals is hampered by three persistent governance challenges that are embedded in the structure of the global system: the sovereignty challenge, the sectoral challenge and the accountability challenge (Frenk and Moon, 2013).

These challenges became painfully tangible during the worst global public health crisis in a century: the COVID-19 pandemic. Chapter 14 shows how achievement of the critical goal of distributing vaccines equitably was subverted by the three governance challenges. Understanding them is therefore not simply a conceptual exercise but an imperative if the world is to do better when the next crisis arrives.

12.2.1 The Sovereignty Challenge

In a world of sovereign nation states, health continues to be primarily a national responsibility. However, the intensified transfer of health risks across borders means that the determinants of health and the means to fulfill that responsibility lie increasingly beyond the control of any one nation state (Jamison et al., 1998). In the absence of a world government, there is an inherent tension between the reality of national sovereignty and the imperative of international collective action to properly manage interdependence. State sovereignty can be critical for protecting public health, for example, when governments need to regulate the practices of multinational firms operating within their borders. But sovereignty can also confound attempts at transnational coordination, rule-making and adjudication. These tasks become even more difficult given the highly unequal distribution of health risks and resources, the opposing interests of various actors, the diversity of cultures and histories and the rapidly changing distribution of power among countries in the global system. For example, competition between sovereign states to secure scarce supplies of COVID-19 vaccines when they first became available in late 2020 meant that many countries had to go without until the needs of more powerful countries had fully been met (Yamey et al., 2022). In a context of deepening health interdependence, it becomes more urgent and yet more difficult for countries to agree on their respective responsibilities, obligations, rights and duties, hampering effective responses to shared health threats.

12.2.2 The Sectoral Challenge

Global health is increasingly the product of cross-sectoral interdependence – that is, the outcome of policy-making processes across multiple sectors (Commission on Social

Determinants of Health, 2008; Kickbusch and Gleicher, 2011). However, the ability of global health actors to ensure that health concerns are adequately taken into account in crucial policy-making arenas such as trade, investment, security, the environment, migration and education remains inadequate. At the same time, COVID-19 demonstrated how profoundly a health crisis can affect the economy, domestic and international politics and human and national security.

12.2.3 The Accountability Challenge

The formal institutions of global governance, such as the United Nations system, are built on the principle that governments of nation states are the primary decision-makers and representatives of their population's interests at the international level. However, new forms of social organization are challenging the primacy of the nation state in the global arena through what David Fidler has called the "unstructured plurality" of non-State actors (Fidler, 2007). For example, civil society networks, experts, foundations, multinational corporations and journalists all wield power in processes of global governance independently of their home-country governments. Two types of accountability problems arise in the current context. The first relates to the legitimacy of intergovernmental organizations, which are formally accountable to the governments of member states rather than directly to the people whose universal rights they are supposed to uphold. This situation too often leads to a "democratic deficit" in the way the organizations operate. This is particularly problematic when people consider their own national governance processes to be illegitimate, such as when governments restrict democratic participation, fail to represent groups that have historically been marginalized or otherwise violate the human rights of their own populations.

The second type of problem is the lack of clear mechanisms for the accountability of non-State actors. The lines of accountability that stretch from intergovernmental organizations to member states to populations are clear, albeit problematic. In contrast, the mechanisms for demanding that non-State actors operating in the global arena – corporations, civil society organizations, foundations, experts and journalists – be accountable for the global effects of their actions are relatively vague, at best. We lack effective institutions to govern the many powerful non-State actors that influence global health today.

These three types of challenges are reflected in efforts to reach international agreement on a new treaty to better govern future pandemics, as illustrated in Box 12.1.

Box 12.1 The Pandemic Agreement: a process riddled with challenges

Since 2021, governments have been negotiating a Pandemic Agreement under the auspices of the WHO. Many countries have been reluctant to agree to strong accountability mechanisms such as independent monitoring, however, out of concerns this could infringe on their freedom of action in the event of a crisis – a clear illustration of the sovereignty challenge. It has also been difficult to reach agreement on the extent to which countries should prioritize controlling diseases that may occur in wildlife or livestock (zoonoses), a frequent source of disease outbreaks in humans; some countries have argued such issues should be addressed by the World Organization on Animal Health or Food and Agriculture Organization, not the WHO – an example of the sectoral challenge at work. Finally, some countries have sought to ensure that private pharmaceutical companies will transfer

Box 12.1 (*cont.*)

technology to enable others to produce vaccines or drugs in the event of a pandemic. However, as international treaties bind governments but not private non-State actors, it has been challenging to agree on ways to ensure this happens – illustrating the accountability challenge vis-à-vis non-State actors at the global level.

After several rounds of negotiations, the Pandemic Agreement was adopted in May 2025 by member states of the WHO. However, the Agreement cannot be opened for signature until an Annex focused on pathogen access and benefit sharing is finalized, which has been a crucial point of tension. As this book went to press, deep divisions between countries remained over the Annex. These challenges reveal how difficult it is to reach consensus on effective rules to govern pandemics at the international level.

12.3 Four Functions of the Global Health System

These three governance challenges impede the performance of the global health system, which must carry out several functions to achieve common goals. Here we describe four key functions of the global health system (Table 12.1) and briefly illustrate the ways in which governance challenges can hinder attempts to carry them out.

The first function is the production of global public goods, especially knowledge-related goods (Røttingen and Chamas, 2012). Examples include tools for international standardization (e.g., the International Classification of Diseases), guidelines regarding best practice (e.g., the WHO Model List of Essential Medicines), research and development of new technologies (see further discussion of technologies in Chapter 8) (Stiglitz, 1999) and comparative analyses and evaluation of policies and programs with respect to design and implementation (Moon et al., 2017). The production of global public goods requires sufficient and sustainable resources, which can be difficult to generate when

Table 12.1 Four essential functions of the global health system

Function	Subfunctions
Production of global public goods	Research and development Standards and guidelines Comparative evidence and analyses
Management of externalities across countries	Surveillance and information sharing Coordination for preparedness and response
Mobilization of global solidarity	Development financing Technical cooperation Humanitarian assistance Agency for the dispossessed
Stewardship	Convening for negotiation and consensus building Priority setting Rule-making Evaluation for mutual accountability Cross-sector health advocacy

sovereign states can benefit from investments made by others without contributing themselves (a situation known as free-riding) (Barrett, 2007). Effective governance arrangements among sovereign states, such as core funding for the WHO or binding legal instruments such as the International Health Regulations, may be needed to overcome the free-rider problem and ensure sufficient production of global public goods (Moon et al., 2012).

The second function is the management of externalities to prevent or mitigate the negative health effects that situations or decisions originating in one country might have on others. It involves the deployment of instruments (e.g., surveillance systems, coordination mechanisms and information-sharing channels) that are essential for controlling the international transfer of risks and ensuring a timely response to threats that spread across borders (e.g., drug resistance, pandemics, environmental pollutants and marketing of unhealthful products such as tobacco). However, sovereignty and weak accountability mechanisms make managing externalities difficult. For example, a government may delay the disclosure of a disease outbreak for fear of economic repercussions, or it could refuse to tighten regulations on an industry that pollutes the air or water flowing into a neighboring country. In both cases, there is no supranational body with authority to stop such a government from generating negative externalities.

The third function is the mobilization of global solidarity, which has been the predominant focus of traditional approaches to global health, mostly through the provision of aid. (We use the term "solidarity" in the context of classical sociological theory, rather than of any particular political ideology, to refer to situations of interdependence created by the complex division of roles characteristic of modern societies (Murray and Frenk, 2000). In fact, the term has been used by groups all along the political spectrum.) The need for this function arises from the unequal distribution of both health problems and the resources to address them. The broad concept of solidarity encompasses four major subfunctions: development financing; technical cooperation, including capacity strengthening; humanitarian assistance to provide relief during natural or human-made disasters; and agency for the dispossessed, in which the global community takes responsibility for protecting the rights of specific groups (e.g., displaced populations or minorities) when their own governments are not willing or able to do so (Jamison et al., 1998). There is a clear case for global solidarity when the health system of a country is chronically incapable of addressing the needs of its population or when it is acutely overwhelmed by a crisis.

The three different framings of global financial transfers for health – development aid, international cooperation and global solidarity – each imply a different set of relationships, types of actors, motivations and instruments (Table 12.2). Although there is not necessarily a linear progression from aid to cooperation to solidarity (in fact, nowadays all three framings operate simultaneously), we argue that the term solidarity not only offers a more symmetrical expression of mutual respect between members of a society but also best corresponds to the underlying conditions of interdependence in an unequal world.

However, carrying out this function can be difficult in a system of sovereign states with few accountability mechanisms. For example, if a state blocks the global community from intervening in the mistreatment of groups that have historically been marginalized under its control, or if it chooses not to contribute to international humanitarian relief efforts, there are few options to make that state do otherwise. Even if a state

Table 12.2 Alternative framings of international financial transfers for health

	Development aid	International cooperation	Global solidarity
Relationship	Dependence	Independence	Interdependence
Actors	Donors and recipients	Independent member states	Members of global community
Motivation	Charity; self-interest	Mutual benefit	Shared responsibility
Main instrument	Discretionary allocations	Pooled resources	Shared resources based on universal rights and duties

commits to providing development assistance, there are few mechanisms for accountability if it reneges.

The fourth function is stewardship, which provides overall strategic direction to the global health system so that all other functions can be performed adequately (Murray and Frenk, 2000). Stewardship includes the following subfunctions: convening for negotiation and consensus building (e.g., regarding policy frameworks such as Health for All through primary health care), setting priorities (e.g., among disease categories or intervention strategies), rule-making to manage the many dimensions of health interdependence (e.g., through the Framework Convention on Tobacco Control), evaluating actors and actions to ensure mutual accountability and advocating for health across sectors. This last subfunction requires health actors to manage the sectoral challenge by learning to advocate effectively for health considerations in the other policy arenas that influence global health. Stewardship requires trusted leadership, legitimate processes and sufficient political space to protect public health in the face of powerful competing interests. Yet all these factors can be undermined when mechanisms for accountability are weak or when sovereign states put narrowly conceived self-interests before global health.

Chapter 14 gives specific examples of how the four functions of the global health system were exercised to face the COVID-19 pandemic.

12.4 Governance of Health Interdependence

Fulfillment of these functions at the transnational level will, in most cases, require building more robust transnational institutions for pooling risks, resources and responsibilities among sovereign states – and in many cases, also non-State actors. Such institutions must deepen cooperation to make it more reliable and to meet the needs of all countries, even if some states might face short-term costs to build more politically sustainable transnational institutions in the long term. For example, states could face immediate economic or political costs by swiftly reporting outbreaks of communicable disease to the WHO, as they are required to do by the International Health Regulations (World Health Organization, 2005, 2020). Other states may face strong political pressure to overreact with counterproductive trade and travel restrictions. Ensuring health security requires rules and compliance arrangements so that states accept costs in the short term, in order to meet their needs in the long term (Moon and Kickbusch, 2021).

But will states share their sovereignty in this manner? In the medium term, this may only be realistic within regions or among smaller groups of states with tightly coupled interests or shared identities. Even among such groups, managing competing interests for the good of the collective has required careful calibration and constant political negotiation. For example, in 2020, bilateral efforts to secure COVID-19 vaccines by some of the EU's member states threatened to undermine EU-wide efforts to secure doses for the full bloc.

Yet the reality of health interdependence requires at least some willingness to strengthen transnational governance arrangements if public health is to be protected. COVID-19 has illustrated how profoundly interdependent the health of each country remains on decisions taken elsewhere. One response has been to mitigate this interdependence, for example, by relying less on globalized supply chains for essential health products through investing in national or regional capacities to produce such goods. But as long as people, goods, services, information, culture and knowledge move across borders, health interdependence will remain a reality that must be governed.

In the absence of a single global political authority – not only now but for the foreseeable future – on what principles can such governance be constructed? Is short-term self-interest the only realistic principle on which to construct transnational institutions, or is there a role for more ambitious concepts like global solidarity? An important test case is the international negotiation toward a pandemic treaty (ongoing at the time of writing) that aims to make responses to future pandemics more equitable than witnessed during COVID-19.

The idea may seem somewhat idealistic, but it is partly based on the observation of a growing density of social interactions and the spread of ideas and norms across borders, which raise new possibilities for developing a sense of solidarity between individuals and societies. For example, when a natural disaster such as an earthquake strikes one country, outpourings of international support often follow – not only from governments but also from individuals moved by images in the media, a reflection of dense social relations and a sense of shared humanity across borders. A fundamental question is whether global solidarity can be fostered in a polity where sovereign nation states coexist with expansive social networks transcending national boundaries, marked by both deep inequality and rapidly changing distributions of power.

12.5 Summary

The global health system is the organized social response to the cross-border transfer of health risks and is comprised of actors whose primary intent is to improve health, along with the rules and norms governing their interactions. The system should perform four essential functions: the production of global public goods, management of externalities, mobilize global solidarity and stewardship. However, the ability of the system to do so is impeded by three types of governance challenges – the sovereignty, sectoral and accountability challenges. Protecting public health in a global context of profound health interdependence requires strengthening transnational governance arrangements.

Comprehension and Discussion Questions

- Give an example of a health threat that has become more significant due to globalization. Similarly, give an example of a health opportunity. Choose a health challenge that cannot be managed by a single country alone. In what ways do the sovereignty, sectoral and/or accountability challenges influence how well it is addressed at the international level?

- What are the four essential functions of a global health system, as discussed in this chapter? Provide an example for each of these functions based on your own experience or a health topic of your choice.
- Do you think the current global health system performs those four functions adequately? Why or why not? Use an example to illustrate your point.

Papers from Which This Chapter Is Adapted

Frenk, J. & Moon, S. 2013. Governance challenges in global health. *New England Journal of Medicine*, 368, 936–942.

Chapter 13

The Imperative of Leadership

Learning Objectives

- Discuss and reflect on the role of leadership in driving change in public health.
- Describe leadership archetypes commonly used in the literature.
- Distinguish between leadership and authority.
- Define the practice of leadership in public health.
- Discuss the role of leadership in health systems performance.
- Discuss leadership competencies.

13.1 Introduction

With this book, we aim to propose a clear conceptual framework that can help bridge the gap between ideas and actions. We strongly believe that clear thinking is a requirement for effective action. The ideas discussed in the previous 12 chapters are meant to provide a series of frameworks through which critical public health problems can be understood and ultimately acted upon.

But clear thinking, while essential, is not enough to ensure action. In Chapter 9, we underlined the role politics, power and policies play in our ability to bring about change. In this chapter, we now turn to the essential role individual actors can play as an agent of change for public health.

By building upon the literature on leadership and system dynamics, we draw the contours of a new understanding of leadership in public health, adapted to the challenges of our time.

In this chapter, we first explore various definitions of leadership, before proposing our own definition. We then turn to the importance of leadership in public health, unpacking why it matters and in which context. We finish by discussing whether leadership can be learned, and if so, which competences need to be acquired by public health professionals to become effective leaders.

13.2 Typology of Leadership

Developing leadership skills is becoming essential to the practice of public health. As mentioned in Chapter 9, leadership is, alongside institutions, systems design and technologies (the LIST acronym), essential for health systems improvement. But leadership might also be the most complex component to address.

Even defining leadership is not an easy task. The Cambridge Dictionary proposes no less than nine definitions to explain the verb "to lead," from showing direction, to controlling a group, a country or a situation, to influencing others (Cambridge Dictionary, 2022). In fact, there is a strong tradition of researchers who have attempted to define what exactly constitutes leadership.

In the nineteenth century and early twentieth century, leadership research often focused on the specific traits and innate qualities of individual leaders and "Great men" (seldom women). But starting in the 1950s, researchers started focusing more on the interaction between leaders and their environments, moving away from a top-down, unidirectional view of leadership (Benmira and Agboola, 2021).

Since the 1970s, there has been increasing recognition of the complexity and multidimensionality of leadership, resulting from multiple interactions between leaders, followers and their environment.

In his 1978 book, *Leadership*, the political scientist Burns distinguishes between two types of leadership: transactional and transformational (Burns, 1978).

Transactional leadership is focused on an exchange of power and benefits between leader and employee. Transactional leaders may use processes, supervision and follower performance in their toolbox to influence employee behavior.

On the other end, **transformational leadership**, sometimes called charismatic or visionary leadership, posits that leaders should encourage, inspire and motivate their followers or employees beyond exchanges and rewards. It focuses on intrinsic motivation of followers, by helping them connect to the leader's goals.

Other theories coexist with these two styles of leadership. **Shared leadership**, for example, focuses more on the complex and continuous interactions and relationships between the leader, followers and their environment. This theory emphasizes the role of human relationships, and the participative process through which leaders involve stakeholders in their decision-making process (Costa et al., 2023).

Many more leadership styles can be found in academic literature. In fact, the leadership scholar Warren Bennis once noted that "leadership is the most studied and least understood topic of any in the social sciences" (Bennis and Nanus, 1985).

In addition, there can be ambiguity on exactly who is identified as a leader. In most research studies, leadership focuses on those at the top of organizations. In contrast, adaptive leadership theory (Grashow et al., 2009) proposes to differentiate leadership from authority. In his book, *Leadership without Authority*, Heifetz argues that people described as leaders in organizations are in reality people in positions of managerial or political authority. In fact, he argues, leadership is not only different from authority but can even be in conflict. 't Hart and Uhr have argued similarly that "leader*ship* is a particular set of activities and interactions that people in position and power as well as *other* people engage in" ('t Hart and Uhr, 2008, p. 3, emphasis is ours). In other words, it is possible to be in a position of authority without exercising leadership, and to exercise leadership without holding formal authority within an organization.

In our view, at its simplest, leadership is the ability *to mobilize others to effect change*. In that sense, we align with theories of shared or collective leadership, which posit that leadership is not a personal trait or a leadership style, but a practice exercised at specific moments in time. In this conceptualization, leadership becomes an activity that can be shared and exercised by all affected by a problem, not just those with formal authority.

In this definition, all actors of the health system, not just medical professionals, epidemiologists or the minister of health can exercise leadership and effect change. In fact, in health systems, we can differentiate between four levels of leadership:

international and national levels, where policy decisions are shaped; sub-national level, where policy translation happens; and local level, where policies and practices are implemented (Chunharas and Davies, 2016).

13.3 Does Leadership Matter?

Next, we turn our attention to the role of leadership in public health and health systems. Considering the difficulties to agree on a definition of leadership, and the complexity of health systems we discussed in previous chapters, it comes as no surprise that there is rather scant evidence on the impact of leadership on public health and health systems performance. Nevertheless, some initial findings emerge. First, longitudinal analyses of health system change in specific settings or for specific topics have shown the role leadership plays in bringing about change (Samuels et al., 2017; Gilson and Agyepong, 2018). For example, a study by Samuels et al. (2017) identified leadership as a key driver for achieving positive health outcomes in maternal and child health in Mozambique, Rwanda and Nepal, the three countries that had achieved the greatest reduction in maternal mortality between 1991 and 2010.

Second, there is a clear consensus among experts and practitioners on the role of leadership in health systems performance. In a study conducted in 2021 by the US Agency for Healthcare Research and Quality, a technical expert panel identified leadership *behaviors*, leadership *engagement in quality and performance efforts* and leadership *incentives* as "very important" to high performance (Ridgely et al., 2020). In 2015, a survey conducted in 65 countries as part of the World Health Organization flagship report on participatory leadership for health reached a similar conclusion on the importance of leadership for health systems (Alliance for Health Policy and System Research, 2016).

13.4 Leadership during Crisis

Particular attention has been placed on studying leadership in moments of crises, including health crises (Glenn et al., 2021). Boin and 't Hart argue that crises are particularly complex moments for leaders, because the imperatives brought about by the crisis, such as to alleviate pain, restore order or bypass regular processes to speed up decision-making are at odds with longer-term processes, including reforms, which require the careful crafting of a vision and the mobilization of actors around it (Boin and 't Hart, 2003). Boin et al. (2005) identified five core tasks of leadership during crises: sense-making, decision-making, meaning-making, crisis termination and learning.

Interestingly, while conventional wisdom may suggest that distributed or shared leadership may not function well in a moment of crisis that requires fast decision-making, several case studies have found the opposite. A detailed case study of the leadership response in Liberia during the 2014 Ebola crisis found that a distributed leadership approach, strategically engaging stakeholders at all levels and communicating intensively about the crisis, was particularly effective to manage the crisis (Nyenswah et al., 2016). The COVID-19 pandemic tragically revealed the roles individual and collective leaderships play: countries and governments that managed the crisis best were not always those most adequately prepared or with the most resources. In fact, some studies have suggested that the level of government and interpersonal trust may have played a key role in limiting COVID-19 infection and fatality rates, a finding that would suggest that building societal cohesion or creating trust in political leaders could be as important to focus on as designing and implementing public health policies (Rountree et al., 2025). A 2023 scoping review, analyzing 45 scientific articles, identified emotional intelligence, communication skills, responsiveness and preparedness, management skills and teamwork as necessary for good leadership during moments of crisis (Osti et al., 2024).

13.5 The Importance of Leadership in Public Health

This evidence suggests leadership is a key driver in health system performance or health systems reform. The importance of leadership in public health can also be understood through the lens of the discipline itself. We highlighted in previous chapters the difficulty of defining and measuring the object of public health itself (Chapters 3 and 4). We also emphasized stewardship and systemic integration as key functions of health systems (Chapter 7) and detailed the role of politics and governance in health system reform (Chapters 10 and 11). Those elements resonate with several aspects of the leadership literature, outlined below.

13.5.1 Public Health Problems as "Wicked" Problems

Many public health problems are classic examples of wicked problems, a key concept for public leadership. The term was coined in 1973 by two urban planning professors, Horst W. J. Rittel and Melvin M. Webber (Horst and Webber, 1973). The authors describe wicked problems as problems that are not easily defined, have innumerable causes and no obvious right answer. These are problems that a purely science-driven approach cannot easily solve. Instead, they require stakeholders to change their mindsets and behaviors. By contrast, a "tame" or soluble problem can be addressed through technical solutions. For example, going to the Moon, while a complex endeavor, is a technical problem. By contrast, addressing climate change is not: stakeholders disagree on the very nature of the problem; its causes are multiple and truly global; and potential solutions, from green technologies to degrowth policies, differ widely.

Contemporary public health issues often contain both technical and wicked components. For example, an epidemic outbreak requires a focus on providing technical solutions (e.g., developing new medicines or vaccines) as well as addressing wicked problems, such as misinformation, community beliefs or power dynamics. This was evident during the COVID-19 pandemic, where challenges such as vaccine hesitancy, or distrust of public health institutions, needed to be explicitly considered to address the crisis.

13.5.2 Public Health Problems as Interconnected Problems

Public health problems are also growing increasingly complex and interconnected, as illustrated in dire terms by the COVID-19 pandemic. The crisis was not merely a health one, but also an economic, educational, social and cultural one: Should governments maintain widespread lockdown or allow children to attend schools? Close borders to prevent transmission or keep them open to facilitate travel or trade? Leverage citizen's private data to facilitate contact tracing or consider their data off limits for such purposes? While all these decisions ultimately related to public health, they required an ability to weigh costs and benefits across multiple sectors with a level of understanding and knowledge that no single individual is likely to possess. They also required stakeholders to efficiently work together to find transversal solutions through collaborations. Similar considerations are at stake when considering the impact of climate change on health. In many ways, these challenges are not different from ongoing discussions on the "polycrisis," a term initially coined by the French theorist of complexity Edgar Morin, recently popularized by the historian Adam Tooze, which describes a state where interconnected and interdependent crises emerge and amplify each other (Delannoy et al., 2025).

13.5.3 Public Health Problems as Political Problems

Finally, public health problems are almost always political, that is, they are concerned with the management and governance of human affairs. This requires those engaged in public health to constantly manage the complex interaction of technical and political work, of scientific evidence and politics. Public decision-making, required to implement population-level policies, involves elements that often go beyond the simple use of scientific evidence to assess impact. This can place public health professionals in a bind: if they remove themselves from the politics, they may become trapped in their role as "technical experts" and lose their ability to influence decisions, leaving the space open for other actors to instrumentalize public health decisions for their own political gains. For example, vaccine hesitancy and refusal prior to and during the COVID-19 pandemic has been linked with populist political rhetoric (Broniatowski et al., 2020; COVID-19 National Preparedness Collaborators, 2022). Studies have shown that the 2014 Ebola crisis played a role during the US 2014 mid-term elections as fears were instrumentalized by political candidates (SteelFisher et al., 2015).

On the other hand, if they become too enmeshed in the political decision-making process, they may lose the credibility as apolitical technical experts that is often the basis for their authority in the first place (Greer et al., 2017). In order to be effective, public health leaders must learn to navigate this paradox and combine evidence-based policy and political skills to achieve the impact they desire.

In this new landscape, public health actors need to successfully influence stakeholders, build coalitions with a wide range of actors and learn to navigate political arenas. Going back to our earlier definition of leadership, they need to mobilize others to effect change.

In conclusion, the nature of public health itself makes leadership critical to its practice. In other words, without leaders, even the best-designed health systems will fail.

13.6 Can Leadership Be Learned?

Before mapping out the components of a leadership practice for public health, we first need to ask ourselves whether those abilities and skills can be acquired. In other words, can leadership be learned?

In her 2006 book, *Mindset*, the psychologist Carole S. Dweck distinguishes between two concepts: the fixed mindset and the growth mindset (Dweck, 2006). Those with a fixed mindset believe that natural abilities are set at birth and cannot be further developed. This is the idea behind the concept of "natural born leaders." To the contrary, those with a growth mindset believe abilities, including personal traits such as courage, creativity or extraversion, can be developed.

Box 13.1 Practicing leadership: the self, the group, the institution

- **The self:** At the individual level, those involved in public health need to become aware of their values, goals, and loyalties, but also their fears and "immunity to change" to develop self-awareness and learn to manage their limitations (Kegan and Lahey, 2016). Practices focused on becoming more centered and "whole" can help public health actors develop clarity on their goals and find more authentic leadership styles.
- **The group:** In groups, public health actors can strive to develop their relational awareness, listening skills and empathy, learn to detect and manage the role of power and authority in group dynamics and understand their own positioning within a collective or a system. By better understanding these collective dynamics, public health actors can help promote groups' social and emotional connectedness, acknowledge and transcend deeply rooted inequalities within systems and help stakeholders find resources within themselves to modify their behaviors to create long-lasting change.
- **The institution:** Finally, public health actors need to consider how their legacy transcends their own work and tenure, to become embedded into the fabric of society. By positioning themselves within a continuum of change, actors can protect the beneficial legacies received from their predecessors and transmit them to their successors. Actors need to consider the role they play in these broader institutional structures, to be able to deliberately align their actions and individual contributions with the broader set of shared goals and values that form societies to create long-lasting change.

The current thinking seems to align with the growth mindset approach. In recent decades, a number of training programs focused on public health leadership have sprouted around the world. There is no doubt that similar initiatives exist at international, regional and national levels in many countries. Those training programs often focus on self-reflection, debate with peers and creating spaces to experiment in low-stake situations and reflect from one's failures. Drawing from the leadership, adult development and psychology literatures, we briefly underline in Box 13.1 some of the topics worth considering when developing leadership training or a leadership practice in public health.

13.7 New Competencies for Public Health Leadership

We finish this chapter with an examination of the specific leadership skills and competencies required for public health. Just like for the definition of leadership, there is no clear consensus on which leadership skills matter when it comes to public health.

In the United States, in 1988, the US Institute of Medicine published a report entitled "The Future of Public Health," calling for the establishment of a more efficient, scientifically sound system of practitioner and leadership development in public health (Walker, 1989). This seminal report helped put more focus on defining a competencies framework for public health in the United States, which is regularly updated and revised. Today, following recommendations from experts, the Centers for Disease Control and Prevention (CDC) identify a core set of public health competencies grouped around eight domains, including "leadership and systems thinking." The latter particularly focuses on cross-sector alignment, organizational change, stakeholder management and advocacy.

Chaumont and McDonald (2024) argued that new public health leaders should focus on five new competencies to address the complex challenges of our times. They are:

- **Societal responsibility:** A clear understanding and commitment to health, including beyond one's sphere of concern or responsibility.
- **Systemic wisdom:** The ability to understand how systems work, to inform how health systems can be aligned with broader policy goals.
- **Comfort with uncertainty:** The ability to make consequential decisions with limited scientific evidence.
- **Mastery of change management:** The ability to understand how change will affect stakeholders, and to accompany them to handle this change and the potential losses it may represent.
- **Focus on execution:** The ability to maintain their drive all the way from policy ideas to impact.

Those skills may represent a departure from a more traditional conception of leadership. Nevertheless, we deem them essential to address the complex, multidisciplinary public health challenges of our times.

13.8 Summary

There is a rich scholarship on leadership, often organized around three archetypes: transactional, transformative and shared leadership. In our view, leadership can be understood as a practice, focused on mobilizing others to effect change. As such, it is not restricted to those in positions of formal authority but can be exercised by all stakeholders in the health system.

Evidence is scarce on the role of leadership in health systems performance, but there is a broad consensus from experts that it does, indeed, matter a great deal. Leadership is essential to public health because public health challenges are, by nature, wicked problems, which are becoming increasingly intersectoral, and sit at the intersection of science and politics.

In the last 30 years, many institutions have started providing leadership training to public health actors. Five leadership skills are of particular importance for the public health challenges of the twenty-first century: societal responsibility, systemic wisdom, comfort with uncertainty, mastery of change management and a focus on execution.

Public health actors can acquire leadership skills by focusing on learning and managing themselves, supporting and accompanying groups and stakeholders to work together toward difficult change, and shaping broader systems and institutions to enshrine the actions they promote into institutional practices and culture. Developing leadership skills is essential: without leaders, even the best-designed health systems will fail.

Comprehension and Discussion Questions

- What is the difference between transactional, transformative and shared leadership?
- Do you agree with Carole Dweck that everything can be learned? Why or why not?
- Thinking about the five functions of health systems (financing, provision of services, resource generation, stewardship and systemic integration, Chapter 11), where do you think leadership matters most? Why?
- Which competencies would you add to the five leadership competencies proposed in this chapter?

Section

4

Synthesis and Conclusions

Chapter 14 Applying the Frameworks to the COVID-19 Pandemic

Learning Objectives

- Deepen understanding of key concepts and frameworks described in this book.
- Illustrate how those concepts and frameworks fit together.
- Apply concepts in an integrated manner to real-world health challenges.

14.1 Introduction

In this chapter, we synthesize the material presented throughout the book using the COVID-19 pandemic as an extended illustration. As the greatest shared global crisis since World War II, the pandemic will have directly touched the lives of nearly every reader and can therefore offer an accessible way of understanding some of the concepts and frameworks presented throughout this book.

In the first days of January 2020, the world began to learn about a mysterious new virus first detected in Wuhan, China. The World Health Organization (WHO) informed governments and the public about the unexplained cluster of pneumonia cases in Wuhan and began tracking the rapidly growing number of cases in China and beyond. Within weeks, cases had been detected around Asia, then the world and, on January 30, the WHO declared the outbreak a Public Health Emergency of International Concern (PHEIC) – the WHO's highest level of emergency alert. By March 2020, the WHO director-general began referring to COVID-19 as a global pandemic. Alarmed leaders shut borders, blocked exports of food and medicines, closed schools and businesses and locked down entire societies in an effort to control the pandemic. Hundreds of millions contracted the virus in the months and years that followed, millions died, hospital and health systems buckled and economies collapsed (Singh et al., 2021).

The longer-term effects on physical and mental health, educational attainment, economic development and politics remain to be fully grasped. We do not try to capture here every major facet of the pandemic – an impossible task in one chapter alone – but rather, we use COVID-19 as an example to show how the concepts in this book fit together and how they can facilitate clearer thinking about public health more broadly.

14.2 COVID-19: A Challenge to Public Health as a Field of Research and an Arena for Practice

In the Preface, we introduced public health as an arena of both research and practice, with knowledge a key driver of the field (Figure 0.1). In the COVID-19 crisis, knowledge was one of the most strategic resources for combating the pandemic – from knowledge of the characteristics of the new pathogen, how it spread and what kinds of effects it caused, to knowledge of how to prevent transmission and mitigate illness. Whether through the use of masks, ventilation and physical distancing, or vaccines, drugs and diagnostics, the way in which knowledge was produced, reproduced, translated and utilized shaped how well a society could respond to the pandemic.

Too often, we witnessed distortions and disruptions in this circle of knowledge. Widespread misunderstanding based on misinformation about the virus, and too often intentional disinformation, underscored what a daunting challenge politicized knowledge poses for the effective protection of public health. In many countries, widespread mistrust in traditional sources of authority or in other members of society impeded the uptake of evidence-based strategies such as community-wide masking or vaccination. For example, in Brazil after the regulatory authority had approved a COVID-19 vaccine for use in children in 2021, President Bolsonaro publicly questioned its safety and announced he would not allow his own 11-year old daughter to receive it, exacerbating vaccine hesitancy in a population that had already witnessed rapidly declining childhood immunization rates (Fernandez et al., 2022). When knowledge was not reliably reproduced, translated or utilized, the consequences for public health were profound.

14.3 COVID-19 as a National Public Health Challenge

COVID-19 was also a reminder that health is not a binary concept, but rather can more usefully be understood as the intensity gradient from perfect health to death (see Figure 3.1 in Chapter 3). Some infected individuals felt no or few symptoms, while others became severely ill or died. The longer-term direct health effects of COVID-19, labeled "long COVID," also seem to vary widely in the population, with some suffering debilitating effects for months or years, and others seeming to recover quickly.

The pandemic highlighted the importance of health metrics (see Chapter 4). The ability to detect, count and track infections was critical for mobilizing political action, setting priorities and making decisions on how to manage the emergency. While the headlines were filled with simple measurements such as cases and fatalities, the pandemic also spurred advancements in modeling to measure not only the current health of the population but also possible future states. Measuring the full health effects of the pandemic is likely to require a wide range of metrics to capture its myriad effects, from direct loss of life to impacts on other health conditions as health systems buckled, from long COVID to mental health repercussions.

Similarly, the pandemic illustrated how national public health is deeply shaped by both the health conditions of the population and the organized social response to those conditions (see Chapter 2 and Table 2.1).

Countries with an epidemiological profile that included a large population of older adults (in particular those above 60 years old) and/or high levels of certain chronic conditions, such as heart disease or cancer, faced major risks of severe illness and death.

But we also saw that demographic or biological conditions alone did not determine outcomes, and that the organized social response made a tremendous difference (see Chapters 7 and 9). For example, despite having a large population of older adults, Japan had the lowest death rate from COVID-19 among all 38 Organisation for Economic Co-operation and Development (OECD) countries as of June 2022, a difference credited to its universal health coverage, high vaccination coverage, widespread masking and low obesity rates, among other factors (Matsuyama and Mayger, 2022).

During the COVID-19 pandemic, the organized social response included not only the functioning of health systems but also the provision of social safety net programs such as unemployment insurance, support for children out of school, measures to ensure food security and capable political leadership. It was a reminder that health depends not only on individual susceptibility to disease agents or on the health system but also on a range of proximate and distal determinants, from housing to family dynamics, from working conditions to political institutions (see Chapter 5 and Figure 5.1). A woman unable to distance herself from an abusive partner or infected family member in a crowded home would be at greater risk of poor health during the pandemic than a woman living in better conditions. A worker, such as a bus driver or supermarket clerk, whose economic survival required them to be in daily contact with many people, would face greater potential exposure to COVID-19 than white-collar professionals who could work from home and have essential goods delivered to their door. Understanding that the response to the public health crisis required more than health interventions alone, many governments took emergency measures to strengthen safety net programs such as financial support to the unemployed and to struggling businesses, temporary housing for quarantines and isolation and requirements for workplace protections. For example, a study found that a government program in India providing public work opportunities during the pandemic cushioned workers from the shock of its economic consequences, particularly rural women (Afridi et al., 2022).

COVID-19 demonstrated that the concept of a one-way epidemiological transition that had once been widely accepted had oversimplified a far more complex reality (see Chapter 6). Most obviously, the era of infectious diseases was clearly not over, and the threat of emerging or re-emerging infectious diseases seemed more daunting than ever – in other words, both a "double-burden" and the potential for a "counter transition" were evident in high-, middle- and low-income countries alike. Intensified international trade and travel, urbanization, destruction of ecosystems bringing wildlife and humans closer together and the consequences of climate change are all expected to make the rapid spread of infectious disease outbreaks more frequent than ever. The higher susceptibility of people with underlying health conditions to severe COVID-19 also underscored the reality that communicable and non-communicable diseases are not binary categories, but rather interconnected.

14.4 COVID-19 and the Performance of Health Systems

COVID-19 shed light on how well health systems – and governments and societies more broadly – performed in the face of this unprecedented crisis (see Chapter 9). An in-depth case study is beyond the scope of this chapter, but a simple comparison between the United States and Japan can provide a concise illustration of the concept of performance. First, it may be useful to recall that the performance of health systems should be seen as relative to the resources available (Figure 9.1). We would not expect a country with low financial resources or limited health care infrastructure or personnel to perform as well as a country with much more.

Therefore, for this comparison we examine the United States and Japan because, despite significant differences (see Table 14.1), they are both large, wealthy countries with well-resourced health systems.

Table 14.1 Indicators for the United States and Japan

	United States	Japan
Total population[a]	332 million	126 million
Percentage over 65/80 years old[a]	11.5%/3.7%	28.6%/9.1%
GDP per capita[b]	$63,028	$42,139
Health spending per capita (current prices, PPP)[a]	$11,859	$4,666
Health spending as % of GDP[a]	18.8%	11.1%
Total health and social employment per 1,000 population[a]	62.6	69.8
COVID-19 deaths per million population[c]	3,093	305
Excess mortality as of mid-2022[c]	15%	<1%

[a] Data from OECD for 2020.
[b] The GDP per capita is measured in terms of purchasing power parity (PPP).
[c] Data from Our World in Data for 2022. COVID-19 deaths per million population are cumulative as of 29 August 2022. Excess mortality is calculated as of May 31, 2022, and defined as "cumulative deaths from all causes compared to projection based on previous years" since January 2020.

As shown in the indicators in Table 14.1, the United States had higher gross domestic product (GDP) per capita, health spending per capita and spent a higher proportion of its GDP on health than Japan. The number of health and social care workers per 1,000 people were similar. In principle, Japan would have been far more vulnerable to seeing excess mortality from COVID-19 due to its large population over 65 years, at 28.6% the highest in the OECD (compared to just 11.5% in the United States). If both health systems performed identically, we would expect the United States to see lower deaths from COVID-19 than Japan. However, what we observe is the opposite: the death rate from confirmed COVID-19 cases was about 10 times higher in the United States, at 3,093 deaths per million persons, than Japan at 305. Another indicator of how well a health system performed under the stress of the pandemic is overall excess mortality, since deaths may be caused by both COVID-19 and other conditions whose management is challenged by a strained health system. On this measure the difference between the two countries is even greater, with the United States experiencing 15% higher mortality (cumulatively from the start of the pandemic to mid-2022) than would have been expected based on previous years' trends, while for Japan the figure was less than 1%.

The reasons for these stark differences in performance are complex and will surely be the subject of research and debate for years to come. Some explanations may emphasize characteristics of the health care system, such as health insurance coverage and depth, or accessibility of care (geographic, financial, cultural and/or psychological) (Anderson et al., 2021). Others may point to factors outside the health care system, such as leadership (Forster and Heinzel, 2021) or societal trust (Bollyky et al., 2022). Measures of pandemic preparedness developed prior to COVID-19 did not predict well which countries would fare better or worse (Kentikelenis and Seabrooke, 2022). Research to understand better how the structure and function of a health system shaped its pandemic response will be critical for reform initiatives, including better preparedness for future crises (see also the Final Thoughts chapter).

We should note that Table 14.1 only reflects one out of the five goals of health systems, that is, improving the total level of population health (defined very simply in this case as mortality linked to COVID-19). A more complete investigation would also examine the other four goals (see Chapter 9 and Table 7.2), including the *distribution* of health – that is, how the health effects of COVID-19 fell unequally across different socioeconomic, racial or other groups in a society. In the United States, for example, lower-income groups were found to be at higher risk of COVID-19 mortality (Abedi et al., 2021), and Black, American Indian/Alaska Native and Latino men and women experienced two to four times the level of excess mortality as Whites in 2020 (Shiels et al., 2021). Such an investigation would also seek to assess the level and distribution of the *responsiveness* of health systems to the needs and legitimate expectations of society – for example, how quickly and well did health systems adapt to population fears of nosocomial infection in hospital settings, or mistrust about the safety of vaccines? Was the health system more responsive to elites versus less privileged socioeconomic groups? Ultimately, it will be important to understand how the burden of financing the COVID-19 response fell across different segments of society: for example, who shouldered the burden of paying for masks and diagnostic tests, for hospital care or vaccination during the pandemic? The extent to which these financial burdens fell on individuals or were spread across a society has varied widely across countries. Considering this wide array of factors will be necessary to paint a fuller picture of the quality, efficiency and equity of a health system. It may also reflect how well a society implemented Health in All Policies, such as those relating to unemployment insurance, education and nutrition.

Finally, the pandemic illustrated how public health is co-produced by the population, not determined solely by specialized disease control agencies or the health care system. It raised a number of complex ethical questions. What do individuals living together in a society – whether a local, national or global one – owe to one another? When does the responsibility to protect the health of others, for example, by wearing a mask or getting vaccinated, supersede the freedom not to? When should a government be able to limit the rights of its citizens to move about freely? How should the rights of children or young adults, who were in general less likely to become severely ill, be balanced against the rights of older adults? What should be the value put on mental health versus physical health? When there weren't enough ventilators or vaccines for everyone, which individuals, population groups or countries should get priority, and how should this scarcity be addressed? Societies varied widely in how they responded to these and other ethical questions, and the implications of these decisions and what they revealed about our societies will likely be felt for years to come.

Chapters 10 and 11 focused on how health systems change and can be reformed. The pandemic has opened policy windows for potential reforms in many national health systems, as well as at the global level, but we exclude discussion of such changes here since at the time of writing these processes were nascent. For an illustration of how health systems can change, see the case study of Mexico in Chapter 11.

14.5 COVID-19 as a Global Health Challenge

As detailed in Chapter 2, the meaning of the term "global health" continues to evolve since it started to be used more frequently at the turn of the millennium. Whereas global health was often used to refer to health issues affecting low-income countries or to certain infectious diseases, COVID-19 has provided one of the clearest embodiments of the broader concept of global health presented in this volume: the health of the global population, with a focus on the dense relationships of interdependence that arise with globalization (Frenk et al., 2014). It also clearly illustrated how the frontiers between national public health and global health are increasingly blurred in a time when the global impacts the local and vice versa.

A virus crossing borders via international travel illustrates interconnection. What COVID-19 so clearly illustrated was not simply interconnection, but interdependence – how much countries depended on each other for information on the virus and its variants, for example, or for supplies of food, masks and vaccines. Referring back to Table 2.2, COVID-19 is a clear example of the global transfer of health risks. It is also an example of how interdependence can give rise to health opportunities. To illustrate, evidence on the safety and efficacy of vaccines was generated in clinical trials in several dozen countries, but provided benefits to all countries that could then adopt those vaccines with confidence. In the wake of the emergency, many countries have also seized the opportunity to strengthen local production of vaccines and other health products to decrease reliance on imports and improve health security. The African Union set a goal that 60% of vaccines needed on the continent be manufactured locally by 2040, and dozens of new production initiatives have been established (Sinumvayo et al., 2024).

What has been the organized social response to the pandemic at the global level? As discussed in Chapter 12, the global health system has the WHO and national governments at its core. Indeed, the WHO has arguably never been as central, under scrutiny or important to global health than it was in the COVID-19 pandemic, and it performed many functions required of the global health system. It performed the stewardship function in gathering information from China in the earliest days of the outbreak, sharing it internationally, and making a judgment as to when it constituted a PHEIC. Director-General Tedros Ghebreyesus and other senior WHO leaders continued to play a stewardship role in exhorting governments, private firms, foundations, media, civil society and others to take more decisive action to control the virus' spread. They also convened the research community regularly to share knowledge, help to coordinate at least some aspects of research and to develop scientific consensus on guidelines. The technical normative guidelines that the WHO produced are an example of a global public good that could support the decisions of national health authorities in all countries (The Independent Panel for Pandemic Preparedness and Response, 2021).

The WHO was also criticized frequently during the pandemic and at times undermined. US President Trump announced in May 2020 that the United States would withdraw as a member state due to concerns over its handling of COVID-19, cutting funding from its largest contributor; this decision was overturned when US President Biden took office in January 2021, then reinstated when President Trump took office again in January 2025. The United States' withdrawal illustrates well the sovereignty challenge (see Chapter 12): countries often work together through the WHO to manage shared health threats, but if a sovereign state decides to stop cooperating there are few measures available to make it do otherwise (The White House, 2025).

The WHO was not the only influential global actor during the pandemic. In April 2020, the Access to COVID-19 Tools-Accelerator (ACT-A) was launched as a multi-stakeholder partnership seeking to make access to vaccines, drugs and other health tools globally and equitably available. It was the product of a handful of governments, foundations, private companies and the WHO and, as such, an apt illustration of the pluralistic mix of State and non-State actors that comprise the global health system. Largely a donor initiative, ACT-A mobilized over $20 billion for the procurement of vaccines, drugs, oxygen and diagnostics and related health system investments from 2020 to 2022, with the lion's share of funding going to COVAX, the vaccine-focused pillar. In many ways, its goal to vaccinate first the most vulnerable 20% of the population in all countries – for example, to prioritize an older adult in a developing country over a young healthy person in a richer country – was an ambitious mobilization of global solidarity (World Health Organization, 2022e).

However, the achievement of that goal was severely undermined by the sovereignty, sectoral and accountability challenges highlighted in Chapter 12. By mid-2020, months before it was clear whether any vaccine would be safe and effective, countries that had the financial, industrial or political means to secure vaccines for themselves first had already done so through a mix of advance purchases, export controls and bilateral agreements. High-income countries plus China, India and Russia – middle-income countries with vaccine development and production capacity – had secured enough vaccines to cover their entire populations, sometimes multiple times over, while low- and lower–middle-income countries were left empty-handed (Yamey et al., 2022). While the ethical and logical approach to taming a global pandemic was for countries to cooperate to get as many vaccines out to as many people as quickly as possible, sovereign states instead put their own short-term national interests before global public health. Political leaders faced strong pressure to meet demand for vaccines domestically first, a dynamic likely to recur in future outbreaks. This case provides a stark example of how health remains primarily a national responsibility, while the means to fulfill that responsibility lie increasingly beyond the nation state. In principle, states can cooperate to achieve shared goals such as controlling an infectious disease, but there is little that can be done if one or more states choose not to.

The global disparity in access to COVID-19 vaccines also reflected the sectoral challenge at work. Health officials rarely controlled decision-making in the pharmaceutical industry, or in the trade or security arenas where decisions on intellectual property (IP) rules or export controls were made. An effort to suspend IP rights on COVID-19-related technologies to accelerate their production (the TRIPS "waiver") was stuck in a political stalemate at the World Trade Organization for 20 months; when governments finally reached an agreement in June 2022 on the proposal, it was too little too late, as the agreement did little to expand production, and by then, countries had found other ways to access vaccines and global supply then exceeded demand (Green, 2022).

Finally, the vaccine issue also offered an apt illustration of the accountability challenge – that mechanisms for accountability are weak to non-existent at the international level. In the early months of the pandemic, promises and rhetoric were lofty and bold. For example, in May 2020 the heads of government of Canada, the European Union, France, Germany, Italy and Norway jointly declared that "If we can develop a vaccine that is produced by the world, for the whole world, this will be a unique global public good of the 21st century. Together with our partners, we commit to making it available, accessible and affordable to all." Those commitments were made under a veil of ignorance, as it was not yet clear which countries would be first to develop or produce an effective vaccine, or how long it would take. It was only a few short months later that the global scramble for vaccine access began, leaving lower-income countries behind.

In many cases, the same wealthy countries that had called for vaccines to be equitably shared as global public goods on the international stage were the ones securing their own supply first through direct agreements with pharmaceutical companies. Few measures existed to hold political leaders accountable for these broken promises, beyond public criticism and a loss of trust.

The global health system proved to be inadequate, weak and ill-suited to an interdependent world facing acute health threats. In 2021, governments launched negotiations toward a pandemic treaty under the auspices of the WHO, to better manage this interdependence through clearer, stronger international rules. At the time of writing, these negotiations were not yet complete (see Box 12.1); nevertheless, its outcome may profoundly influence how effectively and how equitably the world can respond to future pandemics.

14.6 Summary

COVID-19 touched the lives of nearly everyone on this interdependent planet. It exposed and often exacerbated divisions in societies at local, national and international levels, and raised profound ethical and political questions. It also made clear the singular importance of public health services, without which societies cannot function. And it reminded us that protecting and promoting public health is a complex and perennial challenge, full of surprises on a constantly shifting terrain of knowledge, values, interests and politics extending far beyond the health sector alone.

In this way, COVID-19 provides an apt focusing lens through which to conclude this book. The daunting complexity of contemporary public health challenges demands, more than ever, the ability to think clearly about them.

Comprehension and Discussion Questions

- Drawing from your own experience, think of a time when knowledge about COVID-19 seemed incomplete, was confusing to you, or was miscommunicated. Where in the "circle of knowledge" would you place this experience: production, translation or utilization?
- What are the four essential functions of a global health system, as discussed in this chapter? Provide an example for each of these functions based on your own experience or a health topic of your choice.
- Which determinants of health most shaped your own risk of exposure to COVID-19? What is one policy from outside the health sector that influenced your health outcome?
- Using the health system framework from Chapter 9, why do you think the United States experienced worse COVID-19 outcomes than Japan? (If you are more familiar with another country, you may replace the United States or Japan with another country.)
- How did COVID-19 illustrate global interconnection and interdependence? Provide one clear example of each, while ensuring you distinguish between the two concepts.
- Based on the concepts in this book, what reforms would you suggest to improve pandemic preparedness at the national level in your country? What changes would you recommend at the global level?

Final Thoughts: Public Health after the Pandemic

Throughout this book, we have proposed a consistent set of conceptual frameworks that can help to understand the multiple and intricate facets of public health as a field of inquiry and an arena for action. Beyond their individual value, the frameworks are most useful when they can be applied in an integrated manner to a specific public health challenge. Chapter 14 illustrated such an integrative approach around the COVID-19 pandemic – so far the most significant public health event of this century. Because of its magnitude and impact, it brought unprecedented attention to the concepts and practices of public health, which stopped being the exclusive domain of specialists and entered the sphere of awareness of ordinary citizens from every corner of the world. In a very real sense, this has been a watershed moment for public health, a critical test of its capacities and limitations and an invaluable opportunity to reflect on its future.

Historically, most major pandemics have been followed by profound social, economic, political and cultural transformations. For example, according to some historians, after the bubonic plague in medieval Europe, the dramatic decline of the peasant population created the conditions for an improvement in their working conditions and living standards, which in turn paved the way to social movements for expanded liberties (Johnson, 2021). As a negative counterexample, the decimation of the Indigenous people of the Americas due to measles and smallpox introduced by Europeans undermined the attempts by colonizers to press native people into forced labor and set the stage for the importation of African slaves, giving rise to horrific dehumanizing abuses and an ever present legacy of racism that continues to this date in many countries (Nash, 2000).

In some cases, pandemics have been directly responsible for the transformations. In others, they have accelerated or magnified trends that were already present. In every instance, though, pandemics have shaped the societies that emerged from the worlds they disrupted. We have every indication that the COVID-19 pandemic is following the same historical pattern, generating societal aftershocks whose effects continue to be felt well after the pandemic itself has ended.

While these medium- and long-term processes unfold, the immediate task is to distill the main lessons from the COVID-19 pandemic regarding the nature of public health challenges facing the world and the way in which national governments, multilateral institutions and other global actors should prepare for and respond to common threats in the future. This discussion will take time to materialize into actionable reforms. But already it is possible to identify a few valuable lessons:

- To begin with, pandemics are not "natural" processes but instead are as anthropogenic as climate change. COVID-19 should be a wake-up call about the need to protect our planet.
- Furthermore, the pandemic has provided a dramatic demonstration that health is not only a consequence of but also a condition for economic growth and prosperity. Sound economic policy should include the protection of population health and the development of well-performing health systems.
- Equally important, the COVID-19 pandemic has revealed and magnified social inequities. In its aftermath, we should elevate the imperative to promote health equity and social justice.
- In addition, the huge variation in the effectiveness of national responses to the COVID-19 pandemic demonstrates that trust in rational, science-based leadership, which provides clear guidance and brings people together, is crucial for effective collective action during moments of uncertainty.
- Finally, the COVID-19 pandemic has brought into sharp focus the shared frailty of humans in the face of common threats. No local response to such threats can be effective without global solutions.

Applying the lessons outlined above will only be possible if societies demand and governments enact fundamental reforms of the national and global systems required to prevent, prepare for and respond successfully to future pandemics and other emerging challenges. Such reforms must be built on a foundation of innovation: technological innovation stemming from basic research; institutional innovation to improve the performance of public health departments, which have traditionally been the most neglected parts of national health systems; and innovation of the rules of global governance to power new forms of international cooperation better suited to the challenges of the twenty-first century and beyond.

As important as pandemic preparedness and response is, it does not encompass the entire public health agenda in need of reform. As the world emerges from the pandemic, renewing public health will depend on our ability to derive, from the rich intellectual traditions that nourish it, the comprehensive innovations that will guide its future. Many such innovations are taking place around the world. Some were already in motion before the pandemic, which served to accelerate them.

It is beyond the scope of this book to review the full array of promising innovations. Instead, we will conclude with a broad perspective on the unique moment of opportunity we have to build a new era in public health, which is made possible by the convergence of six revolutions currently unfolding.

First is the revolution in the **life sciences**, especially in genomics. The speed with which the COVID-19 vaccine, based on messenger RNA technology, was developed is a testament to this revolution. Advances in the life sciences are essential to attain a better understanding about differential disease patterns in a way that generates solutions suited to specific settings, including resource-constrained health systems. Nevertheless, difficult questions remain regarding who can or should benefit from these advances, as illustrated by the inequitable access to COVID-19 vaccines. New institutional arrangements are needed to ensure widespread access to the benefits of this revolution in the life sciences.

Second is the **information and communications** revolution. Information has never been as widely distributed as the internet and social media have made possible, potentially empowering people to be co-producers of their own health by enabling access to knowledge. Such progress is not exempt from challenges such as dis- and misinformation, illustrated by vaccine hesitancy and dissemination of alternative facts during the COVID-19 pandemic. Public health professionals will increasingly play the critical role of curating such information and of building broader societal trust in science, so it can fulfill its potential to protect health. Included in this revolution are the advances in telecommunications, dramatically accelerated by the pandemic, which are opening exciting new avenues for expanding access to health care and public health services by underserved populations. Governing both the potential risks and harms of this Fourth Industrial Revolution, and ensuring equitable access to its benefits, will be a perennial challenge (Schwab, 2016).

Third is the revolution in **complexity theory and systems thinking**. The Foreword to this book by Dr. Gro Brundtland mentioned the increasing complexity of the health challenges our world faces, which span disciplines and sectors. At the same time, this revolution is generating methods that allow us to better comprehend complexity and develop integrative approaches to transform reality. One application of such endeavors will be the design and operation of adaptive health systems that optimize their value to society through improved structures, processes and outcomes.

Fourth is the revolution in **data science**, allowing unprecedented capacity to process large volumes of information, a lot of it in real time, regarding physiological variables, environmental risks and health system transactions. Closely related is the exponential development of **artificial intelligence**, which, if stewarded with appropriate attention to its social and ethical implications, has the potential of accelerating the other revolutions (World Health Organization, 2021c).

Fifth is the **education** revolution, which is being driven by advances in the cognitive sciences, technological innovations allowing for highly interactive modalities of online learning, unprecedented growth in the global demand for higher education and the rapidly changing labor markets requiring continuous learning throughout the entire life cycle.

Last, but certainly not least, there is what Michael Ignatieff has called the **rights** revolution (Ignatieff, 2006), which is turning abstract declarations about human rights into concrete entitlements that people can be empowered to demand. Inclusive democratic governance and science-based public health practice are threatened in many parts of the globe. But the emergence of a strong civil society, such as the rise of youth to fight climate change, are signs of a type of evidence-based and ethically driven activism that is necessary to secure the future of public health. Without sustained advancement in the rights revolution, the fruits of all the other revolutions will only be accessible to some, and there is a risk of widening inequalities and entrenching injustices, rather than addressing them and improving the health of all.

As the next chapter of public health continues to be written, it is our hope that this volume has accomplished its goal of providing solid intellectual foundations that enable the reader to act effectively for the benefit of people across geographies and generations. The concepts we have discussed are not static. The essence of the circle of knowledge is that its application to solve problems transforms reality and therefore compels us to renew our ways of thinking as new evidence constantly emerges through the subtle dialectic between ideas and practice. More than anything else, this book is a call to embrace the notion that clear thinking is essential for effective action. In our turbulent world, knowledge remains the most powerful force for enlightened social transformation.

References

Abedi, V., Olulana, O., Avula, V. et al. 2021. Racial, economic, and health inequality and COVID-19 infection in the United States. *Journal of Racial and Ethnic Health Disparities*, 8, 732–742.

Abimbola, S., Asthana, S., Montenegro, C. et al. 2021. Addressing power asymmetries in global health: imperatives in the wake of the COVID-19 pandemic. *PLoS Medicine*, 18, e1003604.

Adams, J. 2020. Recommendation regarding the use of cloth face coverings, especially in areas of significant community-based transmission, April 3. https://stacks.cdc.gov/view/cdc/86440.

Adisasmito, W. B., Almuhairi, S., Behravesh, C. B. et al. 2022. One Health: a new definition for a sustainable and healthy future. *PLoS Pathogens*, 18, e1010537–e1010537.

Afridi, F., Mahajan, K. & Sangwan, N. 2022. Employment guaranteed? Social protection during a pandemic. *Oxford Open Economics*, 1, odab003.

Agarwal, N., Meena, C. S., Raj, B. P. et al. 2021. Indoor air quality improvement in COVID-19 pandemic: review. *Sustainable Cities and Society*, 70, 102942.

Aidoo, M., Terlouw, D. J., Kolczak, M. S. et al. 2002. Protective effects of the sickle cell gene against malaria morbidity and mortality. *The Lancet*, 359, 1311–1312.

Ainsworth, C. 2023. Tropical diseases move north. *Nature*, November 9.

Albrecht, G. L. & Devlieger, P. J. 1999. The disability paradox: high quality of life against all odds. *Social Science & Medicine*, 48, 977–988.

Alliance for Health Policy and System Research. 2016. Open mindsets: participatory leadership for health. Flagship report. Geneva: World Health Organization Alliance for Health Policy and System Research. https://ahpsr.who.int/publications/i/item/2016-11-17-open-mindsets-participatory-leadership-for-health.

Alvarado, C. 1976. Concepto de salud pública. In Sonis, A. (ed.) *Medicina Sanitaria y Administración de Salud.* Buenos Aires: El Ateneo.

American Medical Association. 2023. Reducing disparities in health care. www.ama-assn.org/public-health/health-equity/reducing-disparities-health-care.

Anadon, L. D., Matus, K., Moon, S. et al. 2014. *Innovation and Access to Technologies for Sustainable Development: Diagnosing Weaknesses and Identifying Interventions in the Transnational Arena.* Cambridge, MA: Sustainability Science Program and Belfer Center for Science and International Affairs, Kennedy School of Government, Harvard University.

Anderson, K. E., McGinty, E. E., Presskreischer, R. & Barry, C. L. 2021. Reports of forgone medical care among US adults during the initial phase of the COVID-19 pandemic. *JAMA Network Open*, 4, e2034882.

Ashton, J. & Seymour, H. 1988. *The New Public Health.* Maidenhead: Open University Press.

Askari, M., Heshmati, J., Shahinfar, H., Tripathi, N. & Daneshzad, E. 2020. Ultra-processed food and the risk of overweight and obesity: a systematic review and meta-analysis of observational studies. *International Journal of Obesity*, 44, 2080–2091.

Aspen Institute. 2017. Glossary for understanding the dismantling structural racism/promoting racial equity analysis. www.safestates.org/resource/resmgr/connections_lab/glossary_citation/RCC-Structural-Racism-Glossa.pdf.

Atun, R., de Andrade, L. O. M., Almeida, G. et al. 2015. Health-system reform and universal health coverage in Latin America. *The Lancet*, 385, 1230–1247.

Bado, A. R. & Sathiya Susuman, A. 2016. Women's education and health inequalities in under-five mortality in selected sub-Saharan African countries, 1990–2015. *PLoS One*, 11, e0159186.

Bailey, Z. D., Feldman, J. M. & Bassett, M. T. 2021. How structural racism works: racist policies as a root cause of U.S. racial health inequities. *New England Journal of Medicine*, 384, 768–773.

Barrett, S. 2007. *Why Cooperate? The Incentive to Supply Global Public Good*. Oxford: Oxford University Press.

Baumgartner, F. & Jones, B. 2010. Punctuated equilibria in politics. In *Agendas and Instability in American Politics*. Chicago, IL: University of Chicago Press.

BBC. 2020. President Trump calls coronavirus "kung flu". BBC News, June 24. www.bbc.co.uk/news/av/world-us-canada-53173436.

Beaglehole, R. & Bonita, R. 2010. What is global health? *Global Health Action*, 3, 5142.

Beauchamp, T. L. & Childress, J. F. 1989. *Principles of Biomedical Ethics*. Oxford: Oxford University Press.

Bennis, W. & Nanus, B. 1985. *Leaders: The Strategies for Taking Charge*. New York: Harper & Row.

Benmira, S. & Agboola, M. 2021. Evolution of leadership theory. *BMJ Leader*, 5, 3.

Berman, A. 2017. Industry, regulatory capture and transnational standard setting. *AJIL Unbound*, 111, 112–118.

Berman, P. 1993. Health sector reform in developing countries: framing the issues. Conference on Health Sector Reform in Developing Countries: Issues for the 1990s, September, Durham, New Hampshire.

Berman, P., Bridget, E. & Ruck, C. 2024. Is there a "public health system"? How can we describe its organization? In Berman, P. (ed.) *Shaping a Pandemic Response: Evidence, Intervention, Politics, Organization and Governance*. Singapore: World Scientific Publications.

Bernhart, M. H., Wiadnyana, I. G. P., Wihardjo, H. & Pohan, I. 1999. Patient satisfaction in developing countries. *Social Science & Medicine*, 48, 989–996.

Bhargava, A., Jamison, D. T., Lau, L. J. & Murray, C. J. L. 2001. Modeling the effects of health on economic growth. *Journal of Health Economics*, 20, 423–440.

Bircher, J. 2005. Towards a dynamic definition of health and disease. *Medicine, Health Care, and Philosophy*, 8, 335–341.

Birn, A.-E. 2005. Gates's grandest challenge: transcending technology as public health ideology. *The Lancet*, 366, 514–519.

Black, D. 1980. *Inequalities in Health: The Black Report*. London: Department of Health and Social Security.

Bloch, S. & Reddaway, P. 1977. *Russia's Political Hospitals: The Abuse of Psychiatry in the Soviet Union*. London: Victor Gollancz & Futura Publications.

Bloom, B. 2005. Public health in transition. *Scientific American*, 293, 92–99.

Bloom, B. R. 2011. WHO needs change. *Nature (London)*, 473, 143–145.

Blum, A. J. & Hotez, P. J. 2018. Global "worming": climate change and its projected general impact on human helminth infections. *PLoS Neglected Tropical Diseases*, 12, e0006370.

Blumenthal, S. J. & Kong, D. S. 2021. Reimagining public health infrastructure in the 21st century. *The Boston Globe*, September 22.

Boadway, R. & Bruce, N. 1984. *Welfare Economics*. Oxford: Blackwell.

Bobadilla, J. L., Frenk, J., Frejka, T., Lozano, R. & Stern, C. 1990. The epidemiologic transition and health priorities. In Jamison, D. T. & Mosley, W. H. (eds.) *Evolving Health Sector Priorities in Developing Countries*. Washington, DC: World Bank.

Bode, I., Huelss, H., Nadibaidze, A., Qiao-Franco, G. & Watts, T. F. A. 2023. Prospects for the global governance of autonomous weapons: comparing Chinese, Russian, and US practices. *Ethics and Information Technology*, 25, 5.

Boin, A. & 't Hart, P. 2003. Public leadership in times of crisis: mission impossible? *Public Administration Review*, 63, 544–553.

Boin, A. 't Hart, P., Stern, E. & Sundelius, B. 2005. Crisis management in political systems: five leadership challenges. In *The Politics of Crisis Management: Public Leadership under Pressure*. Cambridge: Cambridge University Press, pp. 1–17.

Bok, S. 1986. *Secrets*. Oxford: Oxford University Press.

Bok, S. 1995. *Common Values*. Columbia, MO: University of Missouri Press.

Bollyky, T. J., Hulland, E. N., Barber, R. M. et al. 2022. Pandemic preparedness and COVID-19: an exploratory analysis of infection and fatality rates, and contextual factors associated with preparedness in 177 countries, from Jan 1, 2020, to Sept 30, 2021. *The Lancet*, 399, 1489–1512.

Boualam, M. A., Pradines, B., Drancourt, M. & Barbieri, R. 2021. Malaria in Europe: a historical perspective. *Frontiers in Medicine*, 8, 691095.

Bourdieu, P., Chamboredon, J.-C. & Passeron, J.-C. 1991. *The Craft of Sociology*. Berlin: De Gruyter.

Bowling, A. 2005. *Measuring Health: A Review of Quality of Life Measurement Scales*. Maidenhead: Open University Press.

Brachet-Márquez, V. 2001. Ciudadanía para la salud: una propuesta. *Reflexiones Acerca de la Salud en México*, 43–47.

Briggs, A. 1961. The Welfare State in historical perspective. *European Journal of Sociology*, 2, 221–258.

Briggs, N., Weatherhead, J., Sastry, K. J. & Hotez, P. J. 2016. The hygiene hypothesis and its inconvenient truths about helminth infections. *PLoS Neglected Tropical Diseases*, 10, e0004944.

Brock, D. W. 1993. *Life and Death: Philosophical Essays in Biomedical Ethics*. Cambridge: Cambridge University Press.

Brock, D. W. 2010. Ethical issues in the use of cost effectiveness analysis for the prioritisation of health care resources. In Freeman M. (ed.) *The Ethics of Public Health, Volumes I and II*. Farnham: Ashgate Publishing.

Broniatowski, D. A., Quinn, S. C., Dredze, M. & Jamison, A. M. 2020. Vaccine communication as weaponized identity politics. *American Journal of Public Health*, 110, 617–618.

Brooks, H. 1980. Technology, evolution, and purpose. *Daedalus*, 109, 65–81.

Brown, T. M., Cueto, M. & Fee, E. 2006. The World Health Organization and the transition from "international" to "global" public health. *American Journal of Public Health*, 96, 62–72.

Buchmueller, T. C. & Valletta, R. G. 1999. The effect of health insurance on married female labor supply. *The Journal of Human Resources*, 34, 42–70.

Burns, J. M. 1978. *Leadership*. New York: Harper & Row.

Caldwell, J. 1990. Introductory thought on health transition. In Caldwell, J., Findley, S., Caldwell, O. & et al. (eds.) *What We Know about Health Transition: The Cultural, Social and Behavioural Determinants of Health*. Canberra: Australian National University.

Callahan, D. 1973. The WHO definition of "health". *Hastings Center Studies*, 1, 77–87.

Cambridge Dictionary 2022. Leadership. https://dictionary.cambridge.org (accessed 2022).

Campbell, R. M., Pleic, M. & Connolly, H. 2012. The importance of a common global health definition: how Canada's definition influences its strategic direction in global health. *Journal of Global Health*, 2, 010301.

Carr-Hill, R. A. 1992. The measurement of patient satisfaction. *Journal of Public Health Medicine*, 14, 236–249.

Case, A. & Deaton, A. 2015. Rising morbidity and mortality in midlife among White non-Hispanic Americans in the 21st century. *Proceedings of the National Academy of Sciences*, 112, 15078–15083.

Chaumont, C. & McDonald, T. 2024. Leadership for a healthy tomorrow. *Stanford Social Innovation Review*, 23, 57–58.

Chen, L., Bell, D. & Bates, L. 1996. World health and institutional change. In *Pocantico Retreat. Enhancing the Performance of International Health*

Institutions. Cambridge, MA: The Rockefeller Foundation, Social Science Research Council, Harvard School of Public Health.

Chernichovsky, D. 1995. Health system reforms in industrialized democracies: an emerging paradigm. *The Milbank Quarterly*, 73, 339–372.

Chesnais, J.-C. 1992. *The Demographic Transition: Stages, Patterns, and Economic Implications*. Oxford: Oxford University Press.

Chunharas, S. & Davies, D. S. C. 2016. Leadership in health systems: a new agenda for interactive leadership. *Health Systems & Reform*, 2, 176–178.

Cohen, G., Forbes, J. & Garraway, M. 1996. Can different patient satisfaction survey methods yield consistent results? Comparison of three surveys. *BMJ*, 313, 841–844.

Commission on Social Determinants of Health. 2008. *Closing the Gap in a Generation: Health Equity through Action on the Social Determinants of Health*. Geneva: World Health Organization.

Committee for the Study of Nursing Education 1923. *Nursing and Nursing Education in the United States: Report of the Committee for the Study of Nursing Education . . . and a Report of a Survey*. New York: Macmillan.

Coreil, J., Levin, J. S. & Jaco, E. G. 1985. Life style: an emergent concept in the sociomedical sciences. *Culture, Medicine and Psychiatry*, 9, 423–437.

Cornia, G. A., Jolly, R. & Stewart, F. (eds.) 1987. *Adjustment with a Human Face: Protecting the Vulnerable and Promoting Growth*. Oxford: Oxford University Press.

Costa, J., Pádua, M. & Moreira, A. C. 2023. Leadership styles and innovation management: What is the role of human capital? *Administrative Sciences*, 13, Article 47.

Costello, A., Abbas, M., Allen, A. et al. 2009. Managing the health effects of climate change: Lancet and University College London Institute for Global Health Commission. *The Lancet*, 373, 1693–1733.

COVID-19 National Preparedness Collaborators. 2022. Pandemic preparedness and COVID-19: an exploratory analysis of infection and fatality rates, and contextual factors associated with preparedness in 177 countries, from Jan 1, 2020, to Sept 30, 2021. *The Lancet*, 399, 1489–1512.

Coyte, P., Evans, R., Barer, M. & Marmor, T. 1995. Why are some people healthy and others not? The determinants of health of populations. *Canadian Journal of Economics*, 28, 982.

Crear-Perry, J., Correa-de-Araujo, R., Lewis Johnson, T. et al. 2021. Social and structural determinants of health inequities in maternal health. *Journal of Women's Health*, 30, 230–235.

Crutzen, P. J. 2002. Geology of mankind. *Nature*, 415, 23.

Dalsania, A. K., Fastiggi, M. J., Kahlam, A. et al. 2022. The relationship between social determinants of health and racial disparities in COVID-19 mortality. *Journal of Racial and Ethnic Health Disparities*, 9, 288–295.

Dalton, M., Sanderson, B., Robinson, L. J. et al. 2023. Impact of COVID-19 on routine childhood immunisations in low- and middle-income countries: a scoping review. *PLoS Global Public Health*, 3, e0002268.

Daniels, N., Light, D. W. & Caplan, R. L. 1996. *Benchmarks of Fairness for Health Care Reform*. Oxford: Oxford University Press.

DaVanzo, J. 1990. *Household Production of Health: A Microeconomic Perspective on Health Transitions*. Santa Monica, CA: Rand Corp.

Defo, B. K. 2014. Demographic, epidemiological, and health transitions: are they relevant to population health patterns in Africa? *Global Health Action*, 7, 22443.

Delaney, T., Lawless, A., Baum, F. et al. 2016. Health in All Policies in South Australia: what has supported early implementation? *Health Promotion International*, 31, 888–898.

Delannoy, L., Leveugle, J.-C., Maniatakou, S. & Søgaard Jørgensen, P. 2025. More than a buzzword? Mapping interpretations of the "polycrisis". *Sustainability Science*, December 29. https://link.springer.com/article/10.1007/s11625-025-01790-9.

Deming, W. E. 1989. Foundation for management of quality in the Western world. Paper presented at the meeting of the Institute of Management Sciences, Osaka.

Desai, S. & Alva, S. 1998. Maternal education and child health: is there a strong causal relationship? *Demography*, 35, 71–81.

Desalvo, K. B., Wang, Y. C., Harris, A. et al. 2017. Public health 3.0: a call to action for public health to meet the challenges of the 21st century. *Preventing Chronic Disease*, 14, E78.

Dolfman, M. L. 1973. The concept of health: an historical and analytic examination. *Journal of School Health*, 43, 491–497.

Donabedian, A. 1973. *Aspects of Medical Care Administration: Specifying Requirements for Health Care*. Cambridge, MA: Harvard University Press, pp. 58–88.

Donabedian, A. 1980. *Explorations in Quality Assessment and Monitoring*. Ann Arbor, MI: Health Administration Press.

Donabedian, A. 1986. The Baxter American Foundation Prize Address. *Journal of Health Administration Education*, 4, 611–614.

Dubos, R. 1959. *Mirage of Health: Utopias, Progress, and Biological Change*. New York: Harper & Row.

Dubos, R. 1965. *Man Adapting*. New Haven, CT: Yale University Press.

Dweck, C. S. 2006. *Mindset: The New Psychology of Success*. New York: Random House Publishing Group.

Elman, C., McGuire, R. A. & Wittman, B. 2014. Extending public health: the Rockefeller Sanitary Commission and hookworm in the American South. *American Journal of Public Health*, 104, 47–58.

Evans, J. R., Hall, K. L. & Warford, J. 1981. Shattuck Lecture. Health care in the developing world: problems of scarcity and choice. *New England Journal of Medicine*, 305, 1117–1127.

Farmer, P. 2004. An anthropology of structural violence. *Current Anthropology*, 45, 305–325.

Feinleib, M. 2014. *Health Statistics, History of*. Chichester: John Wiley & Sons.

Fernandez, M., Matta, G. & Paiva, E. 2022. COVID-19, vaccine hesitancy and child vaccination: challenges from Brazil. *The Lancet Regional Health – Americas*, 8, 100246.

Ferrari, A. J., Santomauro, D. F., Aali, A. et al. 2024. Global incidence, prevalence, years lived with disability (YLDs), disability-adjusted life-years (DALYs), and healthy life expectancy (HALE) for 371 diseases and injuries in 204 countries and territories and 811 subnational locations, 1990–2021: a systematic analysis for the Global Burden of Disease Study 2021. *The Lancet*, 403, 2133–2161.

Fidler, D. 2007. Architecture amidst anarchy: global health's quest for governance. *Global Health Governance*, 1.

Fidler, D. 2010. *The Challenges of Global Health Governance*. New York: Council on Foreign Relations.

Fidler, D. 2011. Rise and fall of health as a foreign policy issue. *Global Health Governance*, 4.

Fineberg, H. V. 1985. Technology assessment: motivation, capability, and future directions. *Medical Care*, 23, 663–671.

Fink, G., Günther, I. & Hill, K. 2011. The effect of water and sanitation on child health: evidence from the demographic and health surveys 1986–2007. *International Journal of Epidemiology*, 40, 1196–1204.

Fitzgerald, F. T. 1994. The tyranny of health. *New England Journal of Medicine*, 331, 196–198.

Flexner, A. 1910. Medical education in the United States and Canada. *Science*, 32, 41–50.

Forster, T. & Heinzel, M. 2021. Reacting, fast and slow: how world leaders shaped government responses to the COVID-19 pandemic. *Journal of European Public Policy*, 28, 1299–1320.

Fortney, J. A. 1987. The importance of family planning in reducing maternal mortality. *Studies in Family Planning*, 18, 109–114.

Foucault, M. 1973. *The Birth of the Clinic: An Archaeology of Medical Perception.* London: Routledge.

Frederiksen, H. 1969. Feedbacks in economic and demographic transition. *Science*, 166, 837–847.

Freidson, E. 2017. *Professional Dominance: The Social Structure of Medical Care.* London: Routledge. (Original work published 1970.)

Frenk, J. 1979. Salud, educación y medicina: expectativas y limitaciones. *Ciencia y Desarrollo*, 26, 133–138.

Frenk, J. 1988a. La modernización de la salud pública. *Nexos*, February 1.

Frenk, J. 1988b. La investigación en salud pública: una nueva realidad. *Gaceta Médica de México.*

Frenk, J. 1993a. The new public health. *Annual Review of Public Health*, 14, 469–490.

Frenk, J. 1993b. The public/private mix and human resources for health. *Health Policy and Planning*, 8, 315–326.

Frenk, J. 1994. Dimensions of health system reform. *Health Policy*, 27, 19–34.

Frenk, J. 1995. Comprehensive policy analysis for health system reform. *Health Policy*, 32, 257–277.

Frenk, J. 1998. Medical care and health improvement: the critical link. *Annals of Internal Medicine*, 129, 419–420.

Frenk, J. 2006. Ethical considerations in health systems. In Marinker, M. (ed.) *Constructive Conversations about Health: Policy and Values.* Oxford: Radcliffe Publishing.

Frenk, J. 2015. Leading the way towards universal health coverage: a call to action. *The Lancet*, 385, 1352–1358.

Frenk, J., Bobadilla, J. L., Sepúlveda, J., Rosenthal, J. & Ruelas, E. 1988. A conceptual model for public health research. *Bulletin of the Pan American Health Organization*, 22, 60–71.

Frenk, J., Bobadilla, J. L., Stern, C., Frejka, T. & Lozano, R. 1991a. Elements for a theory of the health transition. *Health Transition Review*, 1, 21–38.

Frenk, J., Chen, L., Bhutta, Z. A. et al. 2010. Health professionals for a new century: transforming education to strengthen health systems in an interdependent world. *The Lancet*, 376, 1923–1958.

Frenk, J., Chen, L. C., Chandran, L. et al. 2022. Challenges and opportunities for educating health professionals after the COVID-19 pandemic. *The Lancet*, 400, 1539–1556.

Frenk, J. & Donabedian, A. 1987. State intervention in medical care: types, trends and variables. *Health Policy and Planning*, 2, 17–31.

Frenk, J. & Durán, L. 1990. Investigación en sistemas de salud: estado del arte en México y perspectivas de desarrollo. *Ciencia*, 41 (special issue), 15–25.

Frenk, J., Frejka, T., Bobadilla, J. L. et al. 1989a. *The Epidemiologic Transition in Latin America.* Liege: International Union for the Scientific Study of Population.

Frenk, J., Frejka, T., Bobadilla, J. L., et al. 1991b. The epidemiologic transition in Latin America. *Boletín de la Oficina Sanitaria Panamericana*, 111, 485–496.

Frenk, J. & Gómez-Dantés, O. 2009. Ideas and ideals: ethical basis of health reform in Mexico. *The Lancet*, 373, 1406–1408.

Frenk, J. & Gómez-Dantés, O. 2017. False dichotomies in global health: the need for integrative thinking. *The Lancet*, 389, 667–670.

Frenk, J., Gómez-Dantés, O. & Knaul, F. M. 2019. A dark day for universal health coverage. *The Lancet*, 393, 301–303.

Frenk, J., Gómez-Dantés, O. & Moon, S. 2014. From sovereignty to solidarity: a renewed concept of global health for an era of complex interdependence. *The Lancet*, 383, 94–97.

Frenk, J. & González-Block, M. A. 1992. Primary care and reform of health systems: a framework for the analysis of Latin American experiences. *Health Services Management Research*, 5, 32–43.

Frenk, J. & Moon, S. 2013. Governance challenges in global health. *New England Journal of Medicine*, 368, 936–942.

Frenk, J., Ruelas, E. & Donabedian, A. 1989b. Staffing and training aspects of hospital management: some issues for research. *Medical Care Research and Review*, 46, 189–220.

Frenk, J., Sepúlveda, J., Gómez-Dantés, O., McGuinness, M. J. & Knaul, F. 1997. The future of world health: the new world order and international health. *BMJ*, 314, 1404–1407.

Fried, L. P., Bentley, M. E., Buekens, P. et al. 2010. Global health is public health. *The Lancet*, 375, 535–537.

Gaede, B. & Versteeg, M. 2011. The state of the right to health in rural South Africa. *South African Health Review*, 2011, 99–106.

Gamborg, M., Andersen, P. K., Baker, J. L. et al. 2009. Life course path analysis of birth weight, childhood growth, and adult systolic blood pressure. *American Journal of Epidemiology*, 169, 1167–1178.

Garratt, A. M., Ruta, D. A., Abdalla, M. I., Buckingham, J. K. & Russell, I. T. 1993. The SF36 health survey questionnaire: an outcome measure suitable for routine use within the NHS? *British Medical Journal*, 306, 1440–1444.

Garrett, L. 2007. The challenge of global health. *Foreign Affairs*, 86, 14–38.

Gee, G. C. & Ford, C. L. 2011. Structural racism and health inequities: old issues, new directions. *Du Bois Review*, 8, 115–132.

Gill, A. 2021. *Global Trends Analysis: Aligning AI Governance Globally: Lessons from Current Practice*. Bonn: Development and Peace Foundation. https://healthai.agency/app/uploads/2025/05/GT-A_2021-03_en.pdf.

Gilson, L. & Agyepong, I. A. 2018. Strengthening health system leadership for better governance: what does it take? *Health Policy and Planning*, 33, ii1–ii4.

Gilson, L., Alilio, M. & Heggenhougen, K. 1994. Community satisfaction with primary health care services: an evaluation undertaken in the Morogoro region of Tanzania. *Social Science & Medicine*, 39, 767–780.

Glenn J., Chaumont, C. & Villalobos Dintrans P. 2021. Public health leadership in the times of COVID-19: a comparative case study of three countries. *International Journal of Public Leadership*, 17, 81–94.

Godue, C. 1992. International health and schools of public health in the United States. In Pan American Health Organization (PAHO) (ed.) *International Health: A North–South Debate*. Washington, DC: PAHO.

Goldhill, O., Furneaux, R. & Davies, M. 2021. 'Naively ambitious': how COVAX failed on its promise to vaccinate the world. *Stat News*, October 8.

Gomes Gonçalves, N., Vidal Ferreira, N., Khandpur, N. et al. 2023. Association between consumption of ultraprocessed foods and cognitive decline. *JAMA Neurology*, 80, 142–150.

Gómez-Dantés, O. 2001. Health. In Simmons, P. J. & De Jonge Oudraat, C. (eds.) *Managing Global Issues: Lessons Learned*. Washington, DC: Carnegie Endowment for International Peace.

Grashow, A., Heifetz, R. A. & Linsky, M. 2009. *The Practice of Adaptive Leadership*. Brighton, MA: Harvard Business Review Press.

Green, A. 2022. WTO finally agrees on a TRIPS deal. But not everyone is happy. *Devex*, 17 June, 17.

Greer, S. L., Bekker, M. P. M., Leeuw, E. D. et al. 2017. Policy, politics and public health. *European Journal of Public Health*, 27, 40–43.

Greszczuk, C. 2019. Implementing Health in All Policies. *Lessons from around the World*. London: Health Foundation.

Grosse, S. D., Lollar, D. J., Campbell, V. A. & Chamie, M. 2009. Disability and disability-adjusted life years: not the same. *Public Health Reports*, 124, 197–202.

Gruber, J. & Madrian, B. 1994. Health insurance and the labour market. NBER Working Paper 6762. Cambridge, MA: National Bureau of Economic Research.

Gruenberg, E. M. 1977. The failures of success. *The Milbank Memorial Fund Quarterly. Health and Society*, 55, 3–24.

Hack, M., Klein, N. K. & Taylor, H. G. 1995. Long-term developmental outcomes of low birth weight infants. *The Future of Children*, 5, 176–196.

Hafferty, F. W. 1988. Theories at the crossroads: a discussion of evolving views on medicine as a profession. *The Milbank Quarterly*, 66, 202–225.

Hagen, S., Ivar Øvergård, K., Helgesen, M., Fosse, E. & Torp, S. 2018. Health promotion at local level in Norway: the use of public health coordinators and health overviews to promote fair distribution among social groups. *International Journal of Health Policy and Management*, 7, 807–817.

Hausman, D. M. 2015. Why measure health? *Valuing Health: Well-Being, Freedom, and Suffering.* Oxford: Oxford University Press.

Hedegaard, H., Miniño, A. M. & Warner, M. 2020. *Drug Overdose Deaths in the United States, 1999–2019.* Hyattsville, MD: National Center for Health Statistics.

Heifetz, R. A. 1994. *Leadership without Authority.* Cambridge, MA: Harvard University Press.

Helgesson, G., Ernstsson, O., Åström, M. & Burström, K. 2020. Whom should we ask? A systematic literature review of the arguments regarding the most accurate source of information for valuation of health states. *Quality of Life Research*, 29, 1465–1482.

Hendriks, A. 1997. Council of Europe – Conseil de l'Europe. Convention for the protection of human rights and dignity of the human being with regard to the application of biology and medicine: Convention on human rights and biomedicine. *European Journal of Health Law*, 4, 89–100.

Herrick, C. 2022. Geographic mythology and global health. *Annals of the American Association of Geographers*, 113, 1516–1533.

Hiam, L., Harrison, D., McKee, M. & Dorling, D. 2018. Why is life expectancy in England and Wales "stalling"? *Journal of Epidemiology and Community Health*, 72, 404–408.

Hill, H. W. 1913. *The New Public Health.* Minneapolis, MN: Press of the Journal-Lancet.

Hill, H. W. 1920. *The New Public Health.* New York: The Macmillan Company.

Hinkle, L. E. 1961. Ecological observations of the relation of physical illness, mental illness, and the social environment. *Psychosomatic Medicine*, 23, 289–290.

Hoffman, S. J., Røttingen, J.-A., Bennett, S. et al. 2012. *A Review of Conceptual Barriers and Opportunities Facing Health Systems Research to Inform a Strategy from the World Health Organization.* Geneva: World Health Organization.

Holt, D. H. & Ahlmark, N. 2018. How do we evaluate Health in All Policies? Comment on "Developing a framework for a program theory-based approach to evaluating policy processes and outcomes: Health in All Policies in South Australia". *International Journal of Health Policy and Management*, 7, 758–760.

Horst, W. J. R. & Webber, M. M. 1973. Dilemmas in a general theory of planning. *Policy Sciences*, 4, 155–169.

Horton, R., Beaglehole, R., Bonita, R. et al. 2014. From public to planetary health: a manifesto. *The Lancet*, 383, 847.

Hotez, P. J. 2016. Southern Europe's coming plagues: vector-borne neglected tropical diseases. *PLoS Neglected Tropical Disease*, 10, e0004243.

Hoyert, D. L. 2022. *Maternal Mortality Rates in the United States, 2022.* Hyattsville, MD: National Center for Health Statistics.

Hsiao, W. C. 1992. Comparing health care systems: what nations can learn from one another. *Journal of Health Politics, Policy and Law*, 17, 613–636.

Human Mortality Database. 2023. Life expectancy. Max Planck Institute for Demographic Research (Germany), University of California, Berkeley (USA), and French Institute for Demographic Studies (France). www.mortality.org.

Huynen, M. M. T. E., Martens, P. & Hilderink, H. B. M. 2005. The health impacts of globalization: a conceptual framework. *Globalization and Health*, 1, 14.

Ignatieff, M. 2006. *The Rights Revolution*. Toronto: House of Anansi Press.

Institute for Health Metrics and Evaluation. 2012. *Financing Global Health 2012: The End of the Golden Age?* Seattle, WA: Institute for Health Metrics and Evaluation. www.healthmetricsandevaluation.org/publications/policy-report/financing-global-health-2012-end-golden-age.

Institute for Health Metrics and Evaluation. 2013. *The Global Burden of Disease: Generating Evidence, Guiding Policy*. Seattle, WA: Institute for Health Metrics and Evaluation.

Institute of Medicine (US) Committee on Employment-Based Health Benefits. 1993. Employment-based health benefits today. In Field, M. J. & Shapiro, H. T. (eds.) *Employment and Health Benefits: A Connection at Risk*. Washington, DC: National Academies Press.

Jamison, D. T., Breman, J. G., Measham, A. R. et al. 1993. *Disease Control Priorities in Developing Countries*. New York: Oxford University Press/World Bank.

Jamison, D. T., Frenk, J. & Knaul, F. 1998. International collective action in health: objectives, functions, and rationale. *The Lancet*, 351, 514–517.

Jha, A. K., Larizgoitia, I., Audera-Lopez, C. et al. 2013. The global burden of unsafe medical care: analytic modelling of observational studies. *BMJ Quality & Safety*, 22, 809.

Johnson, C. R. 2021. How the Black Death made life better. Washington University, St. Louis Department of History News. https://history.wustl.edu/news/how-black-death-made-life-better.

Johnson, T. J. 1972. *Professions and Power*. London: Macmillan.

Kapczynski, A. 2009. Harmonization and its discontents: a case study of TRIPS implementation in India's pharmaceutical sector. *California Law Review*, 97, 1571–1649.

Katzmarzyk, P. T., Salbaum, J. M. & Heymsfield, S. B. 2020. Obesity, noncommunicable diseases, and COVID-19: a perfect storm. *American Journal of Human Biology*, 32, e23484.

Kegan, R. & Lahey, L. L. 2016. *Immunity to Change*. Cambridge, MA: Harvard Business Press.

Kelly, M. P., Stewart, E., Morgan, A. et al. 2009. A conceptual framework for public health: NICE's emerging approach. *Public Health*, 123, e14–e20.

Kentikelenis, A. E. & Seabrooke, L. 2022. Governing and measuring health security: the global push for pandemic preparedness indicators. *Global Policy*, 13, 571–578.

Keohane, R. O. & Nye, J. S., 2001. *Power and Interdependence*, 2nd ed. New York: Longman.

Kickbusch, I. & Gleicher, D. 2011. *Governance for Health in the 21st Century: A Study Conducted for the WHO Regional Office for Europe*. Copenhagen: World Health Organization.

Kindig, D. & Stoddart, G. 2003. What is population health? *American Journal of Public Health*, 93, 380–383.

King, G., Gakidou, E., Imai, K. et al. 2009. Public policy for the poor? A randomised assessment of the Mexican universal health insurance programme. *The Lancet*, 373, 1447–1454.

King, N. B. & Koski, A. 2020. Defining global health as public health somewhere else. *BMJ Global Health*, 5, e002172.

Kingdon, J. 1993. *Agendas, Alternatives and Public Policies*. New York: Harper Collins.

Kinney, E. & Clark, B. 2004. Provisions for health and health care in the constitutions of the countries around the world. *Cornell International Law Journal*, 37, 285–305.

Knaul, F. M., Arreola-Ornelas, H., Touchton, M. et al. 2023. Setbacks in the quest for universal health coverage in Mexico: polarised politics, policy upheaval, and pandemic disruption. *Lancet*, 402, 731–746.

Knaul, F. M., González-Pier, E., Gómez-Dantés, O. et al. 2012. The quest for universal health coverage: achieving social protection for all in Mexico. *The Lancet*, 380, 1259–1279.

Kremer, M. 2004. *Strong Medicine: Creating Incentives for Pharmaceutical Research on Neglected Diseases*, Princeton, NJ: Princeton University Press.

Krieger, J. & Higgins, D. L. 2002. Housing and health: time again for public health action. *American Journal of Public Health*, 92, 758–768.

Krieger, N. 1994. Epidemiology and the web of causation: has anyone seen the spider? *Social Science & Medicine*, 39, 887–903.

Kronenfeld, J. 2019. *Underserved and Socially Disadvantaged Groups and Linkages with Health and Health Care Differentials*. Research in the Sociology of Healthcare, Volume 27. Bingley: Emerald Publishing.

Kuh, D. & Ben-Shlomo, Y. 2004. *A Life Course Approach to Chronic Disease Epidemiology*, 2nd ed. Oxford: Oxford University Press.

Kushel, M. B., Gupta, R., Gee, L. & Haas, J. S. 2006. Housing instability and food insecurity as barriers to health care among low-income Americans. *Journal of General Internal Medicine*, 21, 71–77.

Lagomarsino, G., Garabrant, A., Adyas, A., Muga, R. & Otoo, N. 2012. Moving towards universal health coverage: health insurance reforms in nine developing countries in Africa and Asia. *Lancet*, 380, 933–943.

Last, J. M. 1983. *A Dictionary of Epidemiology*. New York: Oxford University Press.

Latour, B. 2018. *Down to Earth: Politics in the New Climatic Regime*. Cambridge: Polity Press.

Lawal, Y. 2021. Africa's low COVID-19 mortality rate: a paradox? *International Journal of Infectious Diseases*, 102, 118–122.

Leavitt, J. W. 1995. "Typhoid Mary" strikes back: bacteriological theory and practice in early twentieth-century public health. *Isis*, 86, 617–618.

Lee, K. & Fidler, D. 2007. Avian and pandemic influenza: progress and problems with global health governance. *Global Public Health*, 2, 215–234.

Lee, K. & Kamradt-Scott, A. 2014. The multiple meanings of global health governance: a call for conceptual clarity. *Globalization and Health*, 10, 28.

Lee, K., Koivusalo, M., Ollila, E. et al. 2009a. Global governance for health. In Labonté, R., Schrecker, T., Packer, C. & Runnels, V. (eds.) *Globalization and Health: Pathways Evidence and Policy*. New York: Routledge Taylor & Francis Group.

Lee, K., Sridhar, D. & Patel, M. 2009b. Bridging the divide: global governance of trade and health. *The Lancet*, 373, 416–422.

Lema, K. & Morales, N. J. 2020. Philippines to use police in house-to-house searches for COVID-19 cases. *Reuters*, July 14.

Lerner, M. 1973. Modernization and health: a model of the health transition. Presented at the Annual Meeting of the American Public Health Association, San Francisco, CA.

Londoño, J.-L. & Frenk, J. 1997. Structured pluralism: towards an innovative model for health system reform in Latin America. *Health Policy*, 41, 1–36.

Lowe, M. & Hardy Havens, D. M. 1998. Privacy and confidentiality of health information. *Journal of Pediatric Health Care*, 12, 42–46.

Luli, M., Yeo, G., Farrell, E. et al. 2023. The implications of defining obesity as a disease: a report from the Association for the Study of Obesity 2021 annual conference. *eClinicalMedicine*, 58.

Lynch, J., Smith, G. D., Hillemeier, M. et al. 2001. Income inequality, the psychosocial environment, and health: comparisons of wealthy nations. *Lancet*, 358, 194–200.

Maani, N., Collin, J., Friel, S. et al. 2020. Bringing the commercial determinants of health out of the shadows: a review of how the commercial determinants are represented in conceptual frameworks. *European Journal of Public Health*, 30, 660–664.

MacMahon, B. 1970. *Epidemiology: Principles and Methods*. Boston, MA: Little, Brown and Company.

Marinho, F. M. , Soliz, P. , Gawryszewski, V. & Gerger, A. 2013. Epidemiological transition in the Americas: changes and inequalities. *The Lancet*, 381, S89.

Marmot, M. & Wilkinson, R. 2006. *Social Determinants of Health*. Oxford: Oxford University Press.

Marshall, T. 1965. *Class, Citizenship and Social Development*. New York: Doubleday Anchor Books.

Mathers, C. D. 2003. *Health Expectancies: An Overview and Critical Appraisal. Summary Measures of Population Health Concepts, Ethics, Measurement and Applications*. Geneva: World Health Organization.

Matsuyama, K. & Mayger, J. 2022. How Japan achieved one of the world's lowest Covid-19 death rates. *Bloomberg.com*, June 18.

Mazzoleni, R. & Nelson, R. R. 1998. Economic theories about the benefits and costs of patents. *Journal of Economic Issues*, 32, 1031–1052.

McCracken, K. & Phillips, D. R. 2017. Demographic and epidemiological transition. In *International Encyclopedia of Geography*. New York: Wiley.

McDonald, T., Nelson, C., Martin, L. T. & Chandra, A. 2020. Don't waste this crisis: how America can begin building a system of health. www.rand.org/blog/2020/05/dont-waste-this-crisis-how-america-can-begin-building.html.

McDowell, I. 2006. *Measuring Health: A Guide to Rating Scales and Questionnaires*, 3rd ed. Oxford: Oxford University Press.

McDowell, I., Spasoff, R. A. & Kristjansson, B. 2004. On the classification of population health measurements. *American Journal of Public Health*, 94, 388–393.

McInnes, C. & Lee, K. 2006. Health, security and foreign policy. *Review of International Studies*, 32, 5–23.

McKeown, T. 1976. *The Modern Rise of Population*. London: Edward Arnold.

McKeown, T. 1980. *The Role of Medicine: Dream, Mirage, or Nemesis?* Princeton, NJ: Princeton University Press.

Mercer, H. 1987. La medicina social en debate. *Cuadernos Médico Sociales*, 42, 5–13.

Milio, N. 1981. *Promoting Health through Public Policy*. Philadelphia, PA: F. A. Davis Co.

Mitchell, J. A. & Perry, R. 2020. Disparities in patient-centered communication for Black and Latino men in the U.S.: cross-sectional results from the 2010 health and retirement study. *PLoS One*, 15, e0238356.

Monheit, G. D. & Pickett, A. 2017. AbobotulinumtoxinA: a 25-year history. *Aesthetic Surgery Journal*, 37, S4–S11.

Montgomery, M. A. & Elimelech, M. 2007. Water and sanitation in developing countries: including health in the equation. *Environmental Science & Technology*, 41, 17–24.

Moon, S. 2018. Global health law and governance: concepts, tools, actors and power. In Burci, G. & Toebes, B. (eds.) *Research Handbook on Global Health Law*. Cheltenham: Edward Elgar Publishing.

Moon, S. 2019. Power in global governance: an expanded typology from global health. *Globalization and Health*, 15, 74.

Moon, S., Bermudez, J. & 't Hoen, E. 2012. Innovation and access to medicines for neglected populations: could a treaty address a broken pharmaceutical R&D system? *PLoS Medicine*, 9, e1001218.

Moon, S. & Kickbusch, I. 2021. A pandemic treaty for a fragmented global polity. *The Lancet Public Health*, 6, e355–e356.

Moon, S., Røttingen, J.-A. & Frenk, J. 2017. Global public goods for health: weaknesses and opportunities in the global health system. *Health Economics, Policy and Law*, 12, 195–205.

Moon, S., Szlezák, N. A., Michaud, C. M. et al. 2010. The global health system: lessons for a stronger institutional framework. *PLoS Medicine*, 7, e1000193.

Morgan, S. G, Bathula, H. S. & Moon, S. 2020. Pricing of pharmaceuticals is becoming a major challenge for health systems. *BMJ*, 368, l4627.

Mosley, W. H. & Chen, L. C. 1984. An analytical framework for the study of child survival in developing countries. *Population and Development Review*, 10, 25–45.

Mosley, W. H., Jamison, D. T. & Henderson, D. A. 1990. The health sector in developing countries: problems for the 1990s and beyond. *Annual Review of Public Health*, 11, 335–358.

Muller, C. 1985. A window on the past: the position of the client in twentieth century public health thought and practice. *American Journal of Public Health*, 75, 470–476.

Murphy, M., Luy, M. & Torrisi, O. 2019. Mortality change in the United Kingdom and Europe. Working Paper 11-19. London: LSE Department of Social Policy.

Murray, C. J. L. 2002. *Summary Measures of Population Health: Concepts, Ethics, Measurement and Applications*. Geneva: World Health Organization.

Murray, C. J. L. & Chen, L. 1991. The health transitions: dynamics and patterns of mortality change. In Cleland, J. & Hill, A. G. (eds.) *The Health Transition: Methods and Measures*. Canberra: Health Transition Centre, National Centre for Epidemiology and Population Health, Australian National University.

Murray, C. J. & Frenk, J. 2000. A framework for assessing the performance of health systems. *Bulletin of the World Health Organization*, 78, 717–731.

Murray, C., Knaul, F., Musgrove, P., Xu, K. & Kawabata, K. 2013. Defining and measuring fairness in financial contribution to the health system. *GPE Discussion Paper Series*, No. 24.

Nash, G. B. 2000. *Red, White, and Black: The Peoples of Early North America*. Hoboken, NJ: Prentice Hall.

National Health and Medical Research Council. 1996. *Promoting the Health of Indigenous Australians: A Review of Infrastructure Support for Aboriginal and Torres Strait Islander Health Advancement: Final Report and Recommendations/ NHMRC Health Advancement Standing Committee*. Canberra: National Health and Medical Research Council (NHMRC).

Njoku, A., Evans, M., Nimo-Sefah, L. & Bailey, J. 2023. Listen to the whispers before they become screams: addressing Black maternal morbidity and mortality in the United States. *Healthcare*, 11, 438.

Nyenswah, T., Engineer, C. Y. & Peters, D. H. 2016. Leadership in times of crisis: the example of Ebola virus disease in Liberia. *Health Systems & Reform*, 2, 194–207.

O'Donnel, G. & Schmitter, P. 1991. *Transiciones desde un Gobierno Autoritario*. Bueno Aires: Paidos.

OECD. 2024. Technology governance. www.oecd.org/sti/science-technology-innovation-outlook/technology-governance (accessed 2024).

Okada, H., Kuhn, C., Feillet, H. & Bach, J. F. 2010. The "hygiene hypothesis" for autoimmune and allergic diseases: an update. *Clinical & Experimental Immunology*, 160, 1–9.

Olshansky, S. J. & Ault, A. B. 1986. The fourth stage of the epidemiologic transition: the age of delayed degenerative diseases. *Milbank Quarterly*, 64, 355–391.

Omran, A. R. 1971. The epidemiologic transition. A theory of the epidemiology of population change. *Milbank Quarterly*, 49, 509–538.

Omran, A. R. 1982. Epidemiologic transition. 1. Theory. In Ross, J. (ed.) *International Encyclopedia of Population*. New York: The Free Press.

Omran, A. R. 1983. The epidemiologic transition theory. A preliminary update. *Journal of Tropical Pediatrics*, 29, 305–316.

Oreskes, N. 2010. *Merchants of Doubt: How a Handful of Scientists Obscured the Truth on Issues from Tobacco Smoke to Global Warming*. New York: Bloomsbury Press.

Ortagus, M. 2020. Update on U.S. withdrawal from the World Health Organization. US Department of State, September 3.

Osti, T., Valz Gris, A. & Corona, V. F. 2024. Public health leadership in the COVID-19 era: how does it fit? A scoping review. *BMJ Leader*, 8, 174–182.

Ottersen, O. P., Dasgupta, J., Blouin, C. et al. 2014. The political origins of health inequity: prospects for change. *The Lancet*, 383, 630–667.

Oxford Learner's Dictionary. 2024. Definition of network effect. www.oxfordlearnersdictionaries.com/definition/english/network-effect?q=network+effect (accessed 2024).

Panjwani, C. & Caraher, M. 2014. The Public Health Responsibility Deal: brokering a deal for public health, but on whose terms? *Health Policy*, 114, 163–173.

Perkiö, M. 2021. How does women's education influence infant survival? A structural equation model using aggregate data from 95 low- and middle-income countries. *International Journal of Educational Development*, 86, 102465.

Pernick, M. S. 1997. Eugenics and public health in American history. *American Journal of Public Health*, 87, 1767–1772.

Pesec, M., Ratcliffe, H. & Bitton, A. 2017. Building a thriving primary health care system: the story of Costa Rica. Case study, Ariadne Labs. www.ariadnelabs.org/wp-content/uploads/2017/12/CostaRica-Report-12-19-2017.pdf.

Phelps, N. H., Singleton, R. K., Zhou, B. et al. 2024. Worldwide trends in underweight and obesity from 1990 to 2022: a pooled analysis of 3663 population-representative studies with 222 million children, adolescents, and adults. *The Lancet*, 403, 1027–1050.

Possas, C. 1989. *Epidemiologia e sociedade: heterogeneidade estrutural e saúde no Brasil.* São Paulo: Editora Hucitec.

Prado, A. M., Pearson, A. A., Mora-García, C. A. et al. 2024. COVID-19 response and maintenance of essential health services in Costa Rica. Exemplars of Global Research. https://assets.exemplars.health/fd9a20fb-4386-00b3-39a1-1737868b44b7/5077c6e3-7bd8-4158-8331-16c1fac3a52d/ECR_COVID_19_Response_Costa_Rica%20Narrative_R3.pdf.

Preston, S. H. 1975. The changing relation between mortality and level of economic development. *Population Studies*, 29, 231–248.

Pruss-Ustun, A., Wolf, J., Corvalán, C., Bos, R. & Neira, M. 2016. *Preventing Disease through Healthy Environments: A Global Assessment of the Burden of Disease from Environmental Risks.* Geneva: World Health Organization.

Putnam, S. & Galea, S. 2008. Epidemiology and the macrosocial determinants of health. *Journal of Public Health Policy*, 29, 275–289.

Rachels, J. 1975. Why privacy is important. *Philosophy & Public Affairs*, 4, 323–333.

Raine, R., Fitzpatrick, R., Barratt, H. et al. 2016. Essay 5. Evaluating health-care equity. *Challenges, Solutions and Future Directions in the Evaluation of Service Innovations in Health Care and Public Health.* Southampton: NIHR Journals Library.

Raphael, D. 2006. Social determinants of health: present status, unanswered questions, and future directions. *International Journal of Health Services*, 36, 651–677.

Rapoport, A. 1968. Systems analysis: general systems theory. *Encyclopædia of the Social Sciences*, 15, 452–458.

Ravinetto, R., Henriquez, R., Srinivas, P. et al. 2024. Shaping the future of global access to safe, effective, appropriate and quality health products. *BMJ Global Health*, 9, e014425.

Rechel, B., McKee, M. & Jagger, C. 2020. *Living Longer, But in Better or Worse Health?* Copenhagen: European Observatory on Health Systems and Policies.

Reiman, J. H. 1976. Privacy, intimacy, and personhood. *Philosophy & Public Affairs*, 6, 26–44.

Ridgely, M. S., Ahluwalia, S. C., Tom, A. et al. 2020. What are the determinants of health system performance? Findings from the literature and a technical expert panel. *The Joint Commission Journal on Quality and Patient Safety*, 46, 87–98.

Riley, J. C. 1990. Long-term morbidity and mortality trends: inverse health transitions. In Caldwell, J. C., Findley, S. E. & Caldwell, P. (eds.) *What We Know about Health Transition: The Cultural, Social and Behavioural Determinants of Health.* Canberra: Australian National University Press.

Riley, J. C. 2005. Estimates of regional and global life expectancy, 1800–2001. *Population and Development Review*, 31, 537–543.

Rodin, J. 2007. Navigating the global American south: global health and regional solutions. Plenary address presented at the University of North Carolina Center for Global Initiatives, April 19.

Roemer, M. I. 1991. *National Health Systems throughout the World.* New York: Oxford University Press.

Roemer, M. I. 1993. The meanings of social medicine and public health. *Scandinavian Journal of Social Medicine*, 21, 63–65.

Rogers, R. G. & Hackenberg, R. 1987. Extending epidemiologic transition theory: a new stage. *Social Biology*, 34, 234–243.

Rosen, G. 1972. The evolution of social medicine. In Freeman, H. E., Levine, S. & Reeder, L. G. (eds.) *Handbook of Medical Sociology.* Englewood Cliffs, NJ: Prentice-Hall.

Rosero-Bixby, L. 1991. Socioeconomic development, health interventions and mortality decline in Costa Rica. *Scandinavian Journal of Social Medicine. Supplementum*, 46, 33–42.

Ross, C. K., Steward, C. A. & Sinacore, J. M. 1995. A comparative study of seven measures of patient satisfaction. *Medical Care*, 33, 392–406.

Rothman, K. J. 1986. *Modern Epidemiology.* Boston, MA: Little Brown.

Røttingen, J.-A. & Chamas, C. 2012. A new deal for global health R&D? The recommendations of the Consultative Expert Working Group on Research and Development (CEWG). *PLoS Medicine*, 9, e1001219.

Røttingen, J.-A., Regmi, S., Eide, M. et al. 2013. Mapping of available health research and development data: what's there, what's missing, and what role is there for a global observatory? *The Lancet*, 382, 1286–1307.

Rountree, L., Tong, G., Bu, F. et al. 2025. Association of COVID-19 outcomes with measures of institutional and interpersonal trust: an ecological analysis using national data from 61 countries. *Scientific Reports*, 15, 26393.

Ruger, J. P. 2006. Toward a theory of a right to health: capability and incompletely theorized agreements. *Yale Journal of Law & the Humanities*, 18, 3.

Ruthen, R. 1993. Trends in nonlinear dynamics. Adapting to complexity. *Scientific American*, 268, 130–140.

Sabatier, P. & Jenkins-Smith, H. 1988. An advocacy coalition model of policy change and the role of policy orientated learning therein. *Policy Sciences*, 21, 129–168.

Sabatier, P. A. 2007. *Theories of Policy Process*, Boulder, CO: Westview Press.

Sachs, J. & Gallup, J. 1999. Geography and economic development. CID Working Paper No. 1. Center for International Development at Harvard University.

Samb, B., Evans, T., Dybul, M. et al. 2009. An assessment of interactions between global health initiatives and country health systems. *The Lancet*, 373, 2137–2169.

Samuels, F., Amaya, A. B. & Balabanova, D. 2017. Drivers of health system strengthening: learning from implementation of maternal and child health programmes in Mozambique, Nepal and Rwanda. *Health Policy Plan*, 32, 1015–1031.

Saracci, R. 1997. The World Health Organisation needs to reconsider its definition of health. *BMJ*, 314, 1409–1410.

Schlaepfer, L., Alagon, J. & Bobadilla, J. L. 1990. Family formation patterns and child mortality in Mexico. Demographic and Health Surveys (DHS) Program, DHS Further Analysis Series, No. 5, March.

Schwab, K. 2016. *The Fourth Industrial Revolution.* Geneva: World Economic Forum.

Schoeman, F. D. 1992. *Privacy and Social Freedom.* Cambridge: Cambridge University Press.

Scruton, R. 1996. *A Dictionary of Political Thought.* London: Macmillan.

Sen, A. 1981. *Poverty and Famines. An Essay on Entitlement and Deprivation.* Oxford: Oxford University Press.

Sepúlveda, J. 2006. Foreword. In Jamison, D. T., Breman, J. G., Measham, A. R. et al. (eds.) *Disease Control Priorities in Developing Countries*, 2nd ed. Washington, DC: Oxford University Press.

Shi, L., Tsai, J. & Kao, S. 2009. Public health, social determinants of health, and public policy. *Journal of Medical Sciences*, 29, 43–59.

Shiels, M. S., Haque, A. T., Haozous, E. A. et al. 2021. Racial and ethnic disparities in excess deaths during the COVID-19 pandemic, March to December 2020. *Annals of Internal Medicine*, 174, 1693–1699.

Shultz, J. M., Sullivan, L. M. & Galea, S. 2021. *Public Health: An Introduction to the Science and Practice of Population Health*. New York: Springer Publishing.

Shuval, H. I., Tilden, R. L., Perry, B. H. & Grosse, R. N. 1981. Effect of investments in water supply and sanitation on health status: a threshold-saturation theory. *Bulletin of the World Health Organization*, 59, 243–248.

Singh, S., McNab, C., Olson, R. M. et al. 2021. How an outbreak became a pandemic: a chronological analysis of crucial junctures and international obligations in the early months of the COVID-19 pandemic. *The Lancet*, 398, 2109–2124.

Sinumvayo, J. P., Munezero, P. C., Tope, A. T. et al. 2024. Advancing vaccinology capacity: education and efforts in vaccine development and manufacturing across Africa. *Vaccines (Basel)*, 12, 741.

Sitzia, J. & Wood, N. 1997. Patient satisfaction: a review of issues and concepts. *Social Science & Medicine*, 45, 1829–1843.

Smith, A. M. 1981. Dignity and medical procedures. *Journal of Medical Ethics*, 7, 88–90.

Smith, R. 2008. The end of disease and the beginning of health. http://blogs.bmj.com/bmj/2008/07/08/richard-smith-the-end-of-disease-and-the-beginning-of-health.

Smith, R. D. 2006. Trade and public health: facing the challenges of globalisation. *Journal of Epidemiology and Community Health*, 60, 650–651.

Soberon, G., Frenk, J. & Sepulveda, J. 1986. The health care reform in Mexico: before and after the 1985 earthquakes. *American Journal of Public Health*, 76, 673–680.

Stahl, T., Wismar, M., Ollila, E., Lahtinen, E. & Leppo, K. 2006. *Health in All Policies: Prospects and Potentials*. Helsinki: Ministry of Social Affairs and Health, European Observatory on Health Systems and Policies.

Starr, P. 1976. The politics of therapeutic nihilism. *Hastings Center Report*, 6, 24–30.

Starr, P. 1982. *The Social Transformation of American Medicine*. New York: Basic Books.

SteelFisher, G. K., Blendon, R. J. & Lasala-Blanco, N. 2015. Ebola in the United States: public reactions and implications. *New England Journal of Medicine*, 373, 789–791.

Steinfels, P. 1973. The concept of health. An introduction. *Hastings Center Studies*, 1, 3–6.

Stiglitz, J. E. 1999. Knowledge as a global public good. In Kaul, I., Grunberg, I. & Stern, M. (eds.) *Global Public Goods: International Cooperation in the 21st Century*. Oxford: Oxford University Press.

Street, R. L., Jr., O'Malley, K. J., Cooper, L. A. & Haidet, P. 2008. Understanding concordance in patient–physician relationships: personal and ethnic dimensions of shared identity. *Annals of Family Medicine*, 6, 198–205.

Sullivan, D. F. 1971. A single index of mortality and morbidity. *HSMHA Health Reports*, 86, 347–354.

Szlezák, N. A., Bloom, B. R., Jamison, D. T. et al. 2010. The global health system: actors, norms, and expectations in transition. *PLoS Medicine*, 7, e1000183.

't Hart, P. & Uhr, J. 2008. *Public Leadership: Perspectives and Practices*. Canberra: Australian National University Press.

't Hoen, E., Berger, J., Calmy, A. & Moon, S. 2011. Driving a decade of change: HIV/AIDS, patents and access to medicines for all. *Journal of the International AIDS Society*, 14, 15.

Taeihagh, A. 2021. Governance of artificial intelligence. *Policy and Society*, 40, 137–157.

Taeihagh, A., Ramesh, M. & Howlett, M. 2021. Assessing the regulatory challenges of emerging disruptive technologies. *Regulation & Governance*, 15, 1009–1019.

Takagi, L. 2023. Japan sets Luxturna, other new prices while cutting selected fast growers. *Pink Sheet: Regulatory News and Insights*, August 29. https://insights.citeline.com/PS148765/Japan-Sets-Luxturna-Other-New-Prices-While-Cutting-Selected-Fast-Growers.

Tantivess, S., Chalkidou, K., Tritasavit, N. & Teerawattananon, Y. 2017. Health technology assessment capacity development in low- and middle-income countries: experiences from the international units of HITAP and NICE. *F1000 Research*, 6, 2119.

Terris, M. 1975. Approaches to an epidemiology of health. *American Journal of Public Health*, 65, 1037–1045.

Terris, M. 1978. The three world systems of medical care: trends and prospects. *American Journal of Public Health*, 68, 1125–1131.

Terris, M. 1985. The distinction between public health and community/social/preventive medicine. *Journal of Public Health Policy*, 6, 435–439.

The Economist. 2018. The next two decades: the price of human lives. *The Economist*, 427, 11.

The Independent Panel for Pandemic Preparedness and Response. 2021. COVID-19: make it the last pandemic. https://theindependentpanel.org/wp-content/uploads/2021/05/COVID-19-Make-it-the-Last-Pandemic_final.pdf.

The White House. 2025. Withdrawing the United States from the World Health Organization. www.whitehouse.gov/presidential-actions/2025/01/withdrawing-the-united-states-from-the-worldhealth-organization.

Thompson, A. G. H. & Sunol, R. 1995. Expectations as determinants of patient satisfaction: concepts, theory and evidence. *International Journal for Quality in Health Care*, 7, 127–141.

Thorvaldsen, G. 2018. *Censuses and Census Takers: A Global History*. New York: Routledge.

Tikkanen, R., Osborn, R., Mossialos, E., Djordjevic, A. & Wharton, G. A. 2020. Taiwan. In Cheng, T.-M. (ed.) *International Health Care System Profiles*. New York: The Commonwealth Fund.

Tulchinsky, T. H. 2018. John Snow, cholera, the Broad Street pump: waterborne diseases then and now. In Tulchinsky, T. H. (ed.) *Case Studies in Public Health*. London: Academic Press.

UCSF Institute for Global Health Sciences. 2021. Mexico's response to Covid-19: a case study. https://globalhealthsciences.ucsf.edu/wp-content/uploads/2024/02/mexico-covid-19-case-study-english.pdf.

Unger, J. P., De Paepe, P., Buitrón, R. & Soors, W. 2008. Costa Rica: achievements of a heterodox health policy. *American Journal of Public Health*, 98, 636–643.

United Nations. 2020. Word population prospects. Department of Economic and Social Affairs Population Division.

United Nations. 2024. World population prospects. Department of Economic and Social Affairs Population Division.

United Nations Committee on Economic, Social and Cultural Rights. 2020. General comment No. 25 (2020) on Article 15: science and economic, social and cultural rights. United Nations, E/C.12/GC/25.

United Nations Environment Programme. 2021. Era of leaded petrol over, eliminating a major threat to human and planetary health. www.unep.org/news-and-stories/press-release/era-leaded-petrol-over-eliminating-major-threat-human-and-planetary.

Vallgårda, S., Nielsen, M. E. J., Hansen, A. K. K. et al. 2017. Should Europe follow the US and declare obesity a disease? A discussion of the so-called utilitarian argument. *European Journal of Clinical Nutrition*, 71, 1263–1267.

Vateesatokit, P. 2003. Tailoring tobacco control efforts to the country: the example of Thailand. In *Tobacco Control Policy: Strategies, Successes and Setbacks*. Washington, DC: World Bank.

Victora, C. G., Aquino, E. M., Do Carmo Leal, M. et al. 2011. Maternal and child health in Brazil: progress and challenges. *The Lancet*, 377, 1863–1876.

Vigo, D., Thornicroft, G. & Atun, R. 2016. Estimating the true global burden of mental illness. *The Lancet Psychiatry*, 3, 171–178.

Vos, T., Lim, S. S., Abbafati, C. et al. 2020. Global burden of 369 diseases and injuries in 204 countries and territories, 1990–2019: a systematic analysis for the Global Burden of Disease Study 2019. *The Lancet*, 396, 1204–1222.

Wainwright, P. 1994. The observation of intimate aspects of care: privacy and dignity. In Hunt, G. (ed.) *Ethical Issues in Nursing*. New York: Routledge.

Walker, B., Jr. 1989. The future of public health: the Institute of Medicine's 1988 report. *Journal of Public Health Policy*, 10, 19–31.

Warin, M., Bombak, A. & George, B. 2024. Injecting care and negotiating pleasures with weight loss pharmaceuticals. *Thesis Eleven*, 183, 49–68.

Weisz, G. & Harper, J. 2024. Investigating the citing communities around three leading health-system frameworks. *Health Research Policy and Systems*, 22, 16.

Welch, W. & Rose, W. 1915. *Institute of Hygiene: A Report to the General Education Board of Rockefeller Foundation*. New York: The Rockefeller Foundation.

Whitmee, S., Haines, A., Beyrer, C. et al. 2015. Safeguarding human health in the Anthropocene epoch: report of the Rockefeller Foundation–Lancet Commission on planetary health. *The Lancet*, 386, 1973–2028.

Wilder-Smith, A. B. & Qureshi, K. 2020. Resurgence of measles in Europe: a systematic review on parental attitudes and beliefs of measles vaccine. *Journal of Epidemiology and Global Health*, 10, 46–58.

World Bank. 1987. *Financing Health Services in Developing Countries: An Agenda for Reform*. Washington, DC: World Bank.

World Bank. 1993. *World Development Report 1993: Investing in Health*. New York: Oxford University Press/World Bank.

World Bank Group. 2014. A model from Mexico for the world, November 19. www.worldbank.org/en/news/feature/2014/11/19/un-modelo-de-mexico-para-el-mundo.

World Bank Group. 2022a. Life expectancy at birth (years). Washington, DC: World Bank Group.

World Bank Group. 2022b. Mortality rate, infant (per 1,000 live births). Washington, DC: World Bank Group.

World Health Organization. n.d. Evaluating properties, effects and impacts of health technology. www.who.int/europe/activities/evaluating-properties-effects-and-impacts-of-health-technology.

World Health Organization. 1946. Constitution of the World Health Organization. *American Journal of Public Health and the Nation's Health*, 36, 1315–1323.

World Health Organization. 1994. *Principles of the Rights of Patients in Europe: A Common Framework*. Copenhagen: World Health Organization Regional Office for Europe

World Health Organization. 2000. *The World Health Report 2000. Health Systems: Improving Performance*. Geneva: World Health Organization.

World Health Organization. 2005. *International Health Regulations*, 3rd ed. Geneva: World Health Organization.

World Health Organization. 2014a. *Smart Governance for Health and Well-Being: The Evidence*. Geneva: World Health Organization Regional Office for Europe.

World Health Organization. 2014b. *Quantitative Risk Assessment of the Effects of Climate Change on Selected Causes of Death, 2030s and 2050s*. Geneva: World Health Organization.

World Health Organization. 2017. One Health. www.who.int/news-room/questions-and-answers/item/one-health.

World Health Organization. 2018. *Multisectoral and Intersectoral Action for Improved Health and Well-Being for All:*

Mapping of the WHO European Region. Governance for a Sustainable Future: Improving Health and Well-Being for All: Final Report. Geneva: World Health Organization Regional Office for Europe.

World Health Organization. 2020. Statement on the Second Meeting of the International Health Regulations (2005) Emergency Committee regarding the outbreak of novel coronavirus (2019-nCoV). www.who.int/news.

World Health Organization. 2021a. *Global Expenditure on Health: Public Spending on the Rise?* Geneva: World Health Organization.

World Health Organization. 2021b. *COVID-19 and the Social Determinants of Health and Health Equity: Evidence Brief.* Geneva: World Health Organization.

World Health Organization. 2021c. Ethics and governance of artificial intelligence for health: WHO guidance. www.who.int/publications/i/item/9789240029200.

World Health Organization. 2022a. *Strong Systems and Sound Investments: Evidence on and Key Insights into Accelerating Progress on Sanitation, Drinking-Water and Hygiene. UN-Water Global Analysis and Assessment of Sanitation and Drinking-Water GLAAS 2022 Report.* Geneva: World Health Organization.

World Health Organization. 2022b. Noncommunicable diseases. Fact sheet. www.who.int/health-topics/noncommunicable-diseases (accessed November 23, 2022).

World Health Organization. 2022c. Global Programme to Eliminate Lymphatic Filariasis: progress report, 2021. *Weekly Epidemiological Record*, 97, 513–524.

World Health Organization. 2022d. *Framework for the Allocation of Limited Malaria Vaccine Supply.* Geneva: World Health Organization.

World Health Organization. 2022e. World Health Organization (WHO) response to the external evaluation of the Access to COVID-19 Tools Accelerator (ACT-A). www.who.int/news/item/21-10-2022-world-health-organization-(who)-response-to-the-external-evaluation-of-the-access-to-covid-19-tools-accelerator-(act-a).

World Health Organization. 2023. Epidemiological fact sheet: HIV statistics, globally and by WHO region, 2023. www.who.int/publications/i/item/WHO-UCN-HHS-SIA-2023-01.

World Health Organization. 2024. Obesity and overweight. Fact sheet. www.who.int/news-room/fact-sheets/detail/obesity-and-overweight.

World Medical Association. 1981. Declaration of Lisbon. EURO. Principles of the rights of patients in Europe: a common framework. www.wma.net/wp-content/uploads/2005/09/Declaration-of-Lisbon-1981.pdf.

World Trade Organization. 2020. Promoting access to medical technologies and innovation: intersections between public health, intellectual property and trade, 2nd ed. www.wto.org/english/res_e/publications_e/who-wipo-wto_2020_e.htm.

Xu, C., Xu, J. & Wang, L. 2024. Long-term effects of climate factors on dengue fever over a 40-year period. *BMC Public Health*, 24, 1451.

Yamey, G., Garcia, P., Hassan, F. et al. 2022. It is not too late to achieve global COVID-19 vaccine equity. *BMJ (Online)*, 376, e070650.

Yamin, A. E. & Frisancho, A. 2015. Human-rights-based approaches to health in Latin America. *The Lancet*, 385, e26–e29.

Zijdeman, R. & Ribeira da Silva, F. 2015. Life expectancy at birth (total). http://hdl.handle.net/10622/LKYT53.

Index

Printed in the United Kingdom by TJ Clays Ltd.